LISTEN TO YOUR HEART SONG: NAVIGATING THE UNEXPECTED

By

Caron Grossman

Published by:
Wildebeest Publishing Company, LLC
Syracuse, New York

Do you have a story to tell? What's your animal spirit? Share it with us. #hellobeesties

You may visit the author's website at www.carongrossman.com

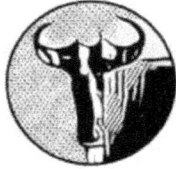

Wildebeest
Publishing Co.

Wildebeest Publishing Company, LLC

For more information about copyrights and usage, special discounts on bulk purchases, workshops, and engagements, please contact Wildebeest Publishing Company, LLC at (315) 220-0217, info@wildebeestpublishing.com, or online at www.wildebeestpublishing.com
Wildebeest Publishing is dedicated to providing flexible remote work opportunities and has a presence in Syracuse, New York City, and Tampa

Wildebeest Publishing Company, LLC paperback and eBook First Edition [February 2025], United States of America

Photograph by Meghan Thomas

ISBN 978-1-958233-36-8 (Paperback Edition)
ISBN 978-1-958233-37-5 (eBook Edition)
LLCN 2024925847

For My Mom
Lydia Deutsch Grossman
6/10/37 - 4/10/77
You mattered
You made a difference
You are loved
Thank you

TABLE OF CONTENTS

CHAPTER 1

ASSESS AND PROCESS

"I'm talking so much my jaw hurts," I laughed, chatting on the phone with my friend, Meg. *What was that twang?* I wondered, as a strange electric current shot up both sides of my jaw. An odd, sharp sensation, perfectly symmetrical, starting at the center of my chin, moving up both sides of my jaw, all the way to my ears. It disappeared as quickly as it came, quieting down to a residual dullness. A minute later, came an ache in my back. It was a subtle, almost imperceptible discomfort. I noted its odd location, not quite between my shoulder blades but two to three inches above, at the base of my neck. I casually mentioned it to Meg, but neither of us gave these twinges a second thought.

After a few more minutes of conversation, I hung up the phone and the discomfort that had settled at the base of my neck had my full attention. I rubbed my neck and shoulders, reaching as far as I could to touch the pain, to massage away what I thought was tension. I twisted and turned my upper body and arms, stretching my back, shoulders, and neck, searching for relief. It didn't feel muscular, but what else could it be? I lay down on my unmade bed, still rumpled in the early morning, and continued stretching, no respite from the slight pain.

Suddenly, my nurse brain kicked in. Sitting straight up at the edge of the bed, I began a head-to-toe assessment of myself. Discomfort at the base of my neck, 2 out of 10. Jaw pain, initially sharp in its quick ascension, now a dull ache, loud enough to remind me it was there. I didn't understand why such vague nigglings held my attention so closely, but I knew I couldn't look away. It seemed impossible for me to think I was having a heart attack; however, I considered taking an aspirin just in case. As I pictured my medicine cabinet, I realized I had none.

A fleeting hope surfaced—*maybe it's just an anxiety attack.* But I knew it wasn't. I anticipated the shallow breaths of an anxiety attack, yet I could pull in an easy breath, deep into my lungs. And I knew I wasn't anxious. In fact, I was incredibly calm.

I continued with my self-assessment. I quickly ruled out a stroke. No facial drooping, my smile was symmetrical, my tongue was midline when I stuck it out, no headache, my arms strong with no drift as I held them out in front of me, as if holding a pizza box. And my thoughts were too clear for my brain to be affected.

I began reviewing the typical symptoms of a heart attack. No shortness of breath. No chest pain or tightness. No numbness, tingling, or pain down my left arm. No sensation of an elephant sitting on my chest. Something was happening, that much I knew, but what? I wanted to rule out a heart attack, too, but I couldn't let it go. I told myself to take another deep breath and mentally step back so I could observe myself more objectively.

I thought of calling Brenda, a cardiac nurse and dear friend. I decided against it, knowing she would tell me to call 911, and I wasn't ready to go down that path. Not yet. Still taking slow, easy breaths, extremely aware of each moment, I had the *brilliant* idea of brushing my teeth, taking a shower, and driving myself to the hospital if this feeling persisted. *It's only two miles down the road*, I reasoned. Fortunately, as quickly as that idea came, it left. It didn't feel wise.

I picked up my pendulum, a simple, clear prism-shaped crystal that hangs at the end of a small chain, gifted to me years ago. Sometimes, I use it to align my intuition with my decisions, asking simple yes or no questions. I watched my back and forth "yes" and the clockwise "no" as it swung in response to my questions. *Is this my heart? Should I go to the hospital?* Both times, my pendulum responded with the back-and-forth motion that indicated "yes." But as much as I enjoyed using my pendulum in making simple decisions I couldn't bring myself to rely on its answers even if it was telling the truth. It was too hard to believe. I didn't want to believe. It was all too outlandish to believe. I wasn't ready to accept what I intuitively knew was happening. Denial can be powerful and, in some cases, deadly.

Still sitting on the edge of my bed, again, I thought of calling Brenda. Again, I decided not to. Instead, I picked up my phone off my nightstand and googled, *Can you have a heart attack after a clean echo?*

After all, it had only been a little over a month since I had a stress echocardiogram, a test using a treadmill and ultrasound that showed how well my heart was working. I received a high five, perfect score, *see you in 2 years* from Dr. Berkery, my cardiologist. This made no sense. How could this be a heart attack? I see Dr. Berkery only because of my family history, not personal history.

I was thirteen years old when my mom died of a heart attack, repeatedly misdiagnosed as having a hiatal hernia. It was almost 45 years ago. She was only 39. Nine years had passed since my dad died of congestive heart failure at the age of 80 after a lengthy history of cardiovascular disease, which included a quadruple bypass when he was 64.

After many years of reckless, unhealthy living, I shifted gears and have done everything in my power to avoid this, working a program of recovery for both food and alcohol, 20 years and 15 years, respectively, tending to my mind, body, and spirit, in the healthiest way possible.

This cannot be my heart, I said aloud to an empty room.

Google said otherwise. Dammit. Reality began to set in.

The word diaphoretic, otherwise known as sweating, unexpectedly popped into my head, another possible symptom of a heart attack. I hoped that my skin would be dry, and I could rule this all out, but as I touched my forehead, the truth of what was happening became clearer as I felt a little sweat. I somehow had the idea that I had time to continue to process because I had no impending doom. No life flashing before my eyes. I was acutely aware of each individual thought that came to me quicker than what I knew time to be. I had never felt so present.

I thought of my adult children, Lindsey and Jake, and wondered, *Is there an age when our kids are old enough for their mom to die?* They may be 34 and 27, but they are still too young to lose me. There's still so much I want to share with them: guidance, unconditional love, accessibility, and presence. They may think they know more than I, but I still have some wisdom to offer, and I love watching them find their way in life.

More importantly, I am not ready to bring this kind of pain to them if I can avoid it. But then I briefly considered, *they will have to deal with it one day anyhow. Why not now? Get it out of the way.* I shook my head vigorously trying to erase the ugliness of that thought like shaking an Etch-a-Sketch.

I thought of Chloe, my eighteen-month-old granddaughter. I want to see her grow up. Who will she become? I want to be a part of her guidance. My kids never had the chance to meet my mom, and I didn't share many stories. I didn't want that for Chloe. There's so much I want to share with her. I want her to know me by our experiences, conversations, and adventures, not by stories and pictures given to her.

I thought of my friends and their reaction if I was to die. I imagined my funeral. Who would be there? What would they say? What would my legacy be? Have I done enough to mean something to each person who showed up? Did my life matter? *Did I matter?*

I thought of dying itself. *Am I ready to die? Do I have any regrets?* I've had a good life, nothing left unsaid. Everyone I love knows that I love them.

The conversation of dying continued in my head, not because it was happening but because I knew I had a choice. If I just lie down, no one would ever know I made the decision on my own. They would just think I had a heart attack. Cardiac arrest. Sudden. Dead.

The movie *Flatliners* flashed in my mind. I remembered how they would bring themselves to the brink of death, extending their cardiac flatline as long as possible before they were brought back to life. I wondered what that would be like. Could I lie down for a bit, get a glimpse of death, and still have time to call 911 if I needed to? How long is too long? What if I pushed it too far and it was too late? If it is my heart, the longer I wait, the more damage to my heart muscle is done. How stupid, selfish, and unnecessary that would be. This wasn't something I could spend time considering. I was alone, and there was no one there to revive me if I laid down too long. Again, I shook my head and moved to the next thought.

I thought about the memoir I've been writing and Wayne Dyer's quote: "Don't die with your music still in you." Am I willing to die before my book is written? The book I have been crafting, in one form or another, for most of my life? I pictured the boxes I have in my closet, filled with journals I've been writing in daily for years. My book may not be assembled, but in many ways, it's already written.

Moving to the next thought, like walking through the cars of a train, I considered the mystery of death—the random thoughts of how and when it will come. The weight of this unknown had been pressing on me more than I realized. For a brief moment, I felt a strange relief, knowing that if I died right here and now, I would be released from that uncertainty forever.

I thought of my mom. At 39, while she lay dying of a heart attack, did she know she had a choice? Or did she believe the doctors who repeatedly told her that her symptoms were a hiatal hernia and would soon pass? The night before she died, she mentioned it again, just before she fell asleep for the very last time.

Mom, Dad, my 17-year-old sister Ellen, me, and even our collie, Timmy, had all climbed onto my parents' bed to watch Saturday Night Live—something we had never done before. Mom had never seen the Coneheads, and she was looking forward to it. To our disappointment, the Coneheads weren't on that episode that night.

"My hiatal hernia is acting up," she said quietly. "I need to go to sleep."

We took our cue and, unusually for us teenagers, recited the mantra of our childhood: "Pleasant dreams, a good night sleep, and I love you very, very much," Mom rolled over to go to sleep, and Ellen, Timmy, and I went off to our own beds.

Sometime during the night, Mom made her way downstairs to the couch in the living room. Did she know she was dying and had laid down too long to change course? Did her life flash before her eyes, or was she fully present, her thoughts clear and concise? Did she have regrets, thoughts and dreams unspoken? At that moment, I felt so close to her, wondering if her experience mirrored my own.

CHAPTER 2

HAPPY EASTER, MY MOM DIED THIS MORNING

As the sun streamed through my living room windows, I was reminded of Easter Sunday, April 10, 1977, so long ago. The memory came rushing back, vivid and unrelenting.

My mom died right in front of me, and I was powerless to stop it. I had heard her making noises downstairs early that morning and thought about checking on her, but it was barely past dawn, and my bed was warm. Then, I heard Dad and Ellen talking in hurried tones. I could hear my dad call an ambulance, giving directions to our home. I rolled my eyes in annoyance, thinking, *No one ever knows where Doll Parkway is.* As concern and curiosity got the better of me, I ran down the stairs.

In the living room, I saw my mom lying on the couch. Ellen held me back at the foot of the stairs in the narrow space between the living room and dining room of our small Cape Cod house. I could see my dad desperately trying to revive her, his voice cracking as he shouted, "Keep her out of here," while he attempted CPR on the soft couch.

I wanted to push past Ellen. I recently learned CPR in school and knew she needed to be on a firm surface. I wanted to scream, *Let me do it. Get out of my way.* But I didn't push. I didn't speak. I didn't move. I stood there paralyzed as I watched the paramedics arrive and take her out the front door on a gurney—the door we used only on Halloween or for special visitors. And they drove away.

People began arriving at the house as we waited for news from my dad at the hospital. The air was thick with fear and uncertainty. I looked around the room. Dad's father and stepmother, Gramps and Aunt Ida, looking small and lost, huddled together on the army green sofa. Mom's friends Marian and Howard Speer arrived. We had dinner at their home the night before, and now here they were, Howard, pacing across the short, green shag rug that stretched from the living room to the dining room. Marian, busying herself in the kitchen. Ellen and I couldn't, shouldn't, be alone as we waited for the phone to ring or Mom and Dad to come home.

I felt confused when Dad finally came home alone—not the dad that had left the house and had gone to the hospital, but this new dad, broken, sobbing uncontrollably, his body shaking with grief. This dad was just as powerless as I was. This dad I saw as weak because he couldn't make it all better. I felt out of my body, observing what felt like a nightmare.

He managed to say the words, "She's dead," as he collapsed into the large orange armchair in the living room. I heard the words, and I knew what they meant, but they made no sense at all. Ellen and I walked over to him, at ages 17 and 13, too large, sat on his lap and cried. We sat there and sobbed with a rawness I had never felt before, keening like an animal that had lost her pup. "She's dead," echoed in my mind, spinning around, trying to find a place to settle.

Eventually, I climbed off Dad's lap, overwhelmed by the enormity of emotions I couldn't begin to process. Everyone around me was crying, hugging, looking around with unfocused eyes. I wanted to run away, scream, make it all go away. I did nothing but stand there and let people hug me until I couldn't take it anymore. I ran upstairs to my bedroom. I threw myself on my bed, crying harder than I had ever cried before until there were no more tears to cry. When I couldn't stand the pain any longer, I escaped outside.

It was a beautiful day. Sunny and warm. One of those perfect Spring days after a long, cold winter that feels so good to be alive. As I walked along the parkway in the middle of my street, bright yellow daffodils were finding their way up through the ground. Mrs. Prahl, my next-door neighbor, was outside and called out, "Happy Easter, beautiful morning today" in that short, polite way that she spoke.

"Happy Easter; my mom died this morning," I replied, continuing down the road, not waiting for a response. I breathed in the sunshine as if all was right with the world.

I gathered up the neighborhood kids, the Powells, the Habibs, and the Prahls, and insisted on starting a kickball game. All the while, I repeated the phrase, as if it fit together like milk and cookies or ham and eggs… "Happy Easter; and my mom died this morning." No one knew how to respond, not just to the tragic and sudden death of my mom but also my reaction to it. I had no answers to the questions they were too afraid to ask, and in my state of shock and denial, all I wanted was to play kickball.

CHAPTER 3

FACING REALITY

I snapped back to the present. No, I don't want Lindsey and Jake's lives flipped upside down with my death, not if I can help it. Thoughts began to emerge, each one clear and precise, like a series of revelations. I was amazed and in awe of just how clear and vivid each thought was.

I thought of how many times I had heard that women present differently than men when having a heart attack. Yet, no one ever specifies what the differences are. What if this is the difference? What if it's as subtle as a swift electric current shooting up the jaw, dulling as quickly as it came? What if it's just an uncomfortable 2 out of 10 ache at the base of your neck, nowhere near where you would think it would be? I glanced around the small room one last time, my senses heightened. The Winter Solstice sunshine poured through the windows, the sounds of cars speeding by on the busy street outside, the aroma of coffee from the mug on the end table. As unbelievable as it seemed, I could no longer deny what was happening.

Somehow, my phone ended up in the middle of my living room floor. I sank to my knees on the soft purple throw rug and, without picking it up, pressed 911 and hit speaker. A man answered, and I calmly said, "I think I'm having a heart attack." I felt a deep surrender in speaking the truth to someone who could take action.

He asked, "Are you having chest pain, pain in your left arm, jaw pain, sweating, shortness of breath?"

"Yes, yes, yes, yes, and yes," I responded, unwilling to admit I had just a dull ache in my jaw and a 2 out of 10 discomfort at the base of my neck. I couldn't take the risk of not being taken seriously. Of not being heard.

He reassured gently, "Someone is on the way," and hung up the phone.

Initial surprise of the abruptness of the end of the call turned to relief. In the movies, they stay on the phone until someone arrives. I called Lindsey, then Meg. No answer. I was grateful they didn't pick up; what would I have told them if they did?

Finally, I called Brenda. She answered quickly, with a sing-song, "Hi, friend."

"I think I'm having a heart attack, and I called 911," I blurted out, feeling a deep release as the tears I didn't know I was holding back began to flow.

"Breathe in through your nose and out through your mouth," She calmly told me. "Slow and easy."

I listened, and I breathed.

"I hear sirens getting closer," I told Brenda, eager for this to move forward.

"Okay, keep focusing on your breath," she encouraged.

"I hear them coming up the stairs," I said as if I was updating her on the news. "I need to let them in," I continued.

"Is your door locked?" she asked as my breathing steadied.

"No," I answered. "But I need to welcome them," attempting to assert some control.

She suggested I stay put and let them come in on their own, but I insisted.

I stood to walk the ten steps to the kitchen door. "I love you," we both said before hanging up.

I had spent 25-30 minutes assessing, observing, processing, calling. Now, I was ready to let others take over. My surrender deepened, and somehow, I knew I would be alright.

CHAPTER 4

SURRENDERING TO THE CARE OF OTHERS

Only four minutes had passed since I called 911 and their arrival. As I opened the door to let the first responders in, I surprised us all by collapsing to the kitchen floor and curled into a fetal position out of complete relief and gratitude for their help. I wasn't thinking how startling falling to the floor would look. Actually, I wasn't thinking at all. All my clear thinking I was in awe of only a few minutes earlier vanished as I handed my care over to them.

The paramedic helped me into a chair, and they quickly went to work, checking vital signs, EKG, three baby aspirin in my mouth, nitroglycerin under my tongue. No one said anything, but I knew. As a nurse, I know the language of this particular silence. Two more paramedics arrived. With COVID masks on, all I could see were eyes. Chris, with her beautiful, clear, gentle blue/green eyes, took over. Her presence was kind, capable, and calming. She held space for me to breathe and trust. I knew my life was in their hands, and I knew I would be alright.

I participated in my care by following all directions, offering up my best vein for an IV, answering every question, remaining calm, breathing. Always focusing on my breath. Chris never took her eyes off mine, yet she moved swiftly and smoothly around the kitchen, placing my phone, charger, hospital ID, and shoes into my large purse.

Two first responders managed to get me down my 15 unusually steep, snowy stairs to the ambulance with a "stair chair," which allows EMS to glide rather than carry down the stairs. I tend to make silly jokes when I am nervous; however, this was the first time I made a little quip because this trip down the stairs, like being at the peak of a roller coaster, just before the drop, was the scariest thing yet.

Another deep breath in, shutting my eyes as I remembered to let go and surrender. I heard them say words of reassurance, words I had said to many patients and families before. Words meant to soothe, whether they are true or not. I chose to believe them as the pain at the base of my neck increased to a 4 out of 10. As Chris called into Crouse Hospital, where I work, to let them know we were on our way, I heard her say STEMI, which means ST-elevation myocardial infarction. A heart attack. An artery is blocked. Shit. Not good at all.

She then said the words, "We are heading in with one of your own."

When I heard that, I felt my surrender deepen. It gave me a strong sense of belonging, of being part of a community, something bigger than I ever knew. This was real. This was happening. We were only two miles from the hospital, sirens blaring. I could picture every stop light, every landmark, knowing the route like the back of my hand from the countless drives to work. The discomfort had become a 5 out of 10. But I had faith in the knowledge and care of others. I knew I would be okay because still, I had no impending doom. Please, just hurry...

It was then, in the back of the ambulance, I remembered to pray. It struck me as kind of funny. As important as my relationship is with my Higher Power, I had been going through this experience for close to 45 minutes and it hadn't crossed my mind to pray. I realize now that I was so present during this entire experience before I handed myself over to others there was no need for prayer. My presence was prayer. When I did finally think to pray, it was no foxhole prayer asking to be saved, just an emphatic, "DUDE (aka, Higher Power), were you not in on the conversation we were just having with Meg this morning? We have big things to do." An odd prayer, to be sure, yet it was a connection, and that was all I needed. Then, any previous thoughts of dying disappeared. I wanted to live.

As we arrived at the hospital through the Emergency Department where I once worked years ago, Mike, an RN I know well, met us at the door. Seeing him, a kind and competent man I have known for 20 years, broke open the dam I thought was fully secured, and again, the tears flowed.

There was a combination of relief and urgency as I looked at him with a mix of confusion and hope and asked, "Mike, what the fuck?"

He gently touched my arm and said, "We've got you, Caron."

I believed him.

The paramedics pushed me on a stretcher, running through the ED to the Cath Lab, not stopping as the person from patient registration yelled out questions, "Any change in insurance or address?"

"No," I yelled back, already 20-30 feet down the hall.

A COVID mask landed on my face, frisbeed over by someone, somewhere, unable to attach to my ears in the hurry.

As we arrived at the Cath Lab, I heard Jo, a cardiac Nurse Practitioner, shouting out consent to me, running alongside the stretcher, going down the list of what was going to occur, along with the risks, and asking if I agreed. "YES!" I said, so grateful that I was being handed off to the next group of skilled and proficient people. The last thing I heard Jo ask was if I consented to receive blood if needed, triggering the urgency of what was happening and what could go wrong. Again, staring up at the fluorescent lights flying by on the ceiling, I said, "YES."

Megan, the manager of the Cath Lab, had been waiting for me and took my hand as I arrived. She, too, said, "We've got you, Caron," with deep compassion in her eyes. I felt so taken care of. Again, I knew I was going to be okay.

As they wheeled me into the procedure room and were about to lift me onto the table, I asked if I could move myself over. I needed to do this. I needed to participate in my care. The sense of power- lessness I felt was huge. I needed some sense of control. I moved myself over to the hard table and laid down on my back as this new group of people, like a choreographed dance, all took their places, all knowing their roles and their marks to stand. There was a quick grace in their movements with little needing to be said.

My right arm strapped down as Dr. George, the same doctor who pronounced my dad's time of death from congestive heart failure nine years earlier, told me what was about to take place. He would be inserting a tiny catheter into my heart through my radial artery. I asked to be knocked out, surprised that I would be staying awake. I figured if they put me to sleep and I didn't make it, I wouldn't know the difference. I didn't want to hear or feel if anything went wrong. Disappointed I didn't get to choose, yet, I trusted the process.

The pain at the base of my neck was now a 6/10. I knew that as soon as the blockage was removed and the artery was opened, I would have relief. I just needed to hang in there until then. I stared at the ceiling, finding a focal point, honing in on my breathing, remembering the many tools I've learned over the years to relieve anxiety.

Then, I heard the word "dissection." Dissection? What's dissecting? My artery? My aorta? My consent to receive blood flashed through my mind, though fortunately, I didn't need it. I knew too much about what was going on, thinking that I just wanted to be knocked out. I didn't want to hear any of this. Fentanyl was ordered for pain that was now 7 out of 10 and given through my IV. Two more doses with no relief. I heard Dr. George ask for John (his partner) to get in there fast to assist with the dissection, all the while calmly asking me if I was okay. As calm as he sounded, there was a quiet urgency filling the room. It was thick and heavy, although I still knew I would be okay, the word "hurry" silently shouted in my head.

Megan saw my face through the glass separating us and asked

for me to receive Versed, a drug that relaxes the body and can induce amnesia. Yes, I thought. Finally, I will sleep.

I heard the nurse say, "One milligram Versed going in," as she pushed the medication through my IV.

I looked at her pleadingly and reminded her, "There are two milligrams in the vial, and I'd like the other, please."

She smiled kindly but didn't give me the second dose. No sleep, relaxation, or amnesia was going to come. After some time, I could feel the tension in the room and in my body subside. And then, as quick as it all started, we were done. The pain was gone.

I could feel the relief fill the room. I was okay.

"Wasting 25 and 1," I heard the nurse say, meaning the medication she didn't use.

With my adrenaline still on overdrive, I reminded her that I was still there, willing to receive whatever was left over.

She laughed as if I told a joke. I wasn't joking.

Before I knew it, I was sitting up on a stretcher, smiling, chatting, and ready to go to my room. It all felt surreal. Less than three hours had passed since I felt the first twinge in my jaw. It was beyond my capacity to process the severity of what occurred. The mood was light and filled with smiles, giving no hint that everything could've looked very different. I took one more deep breath and called my kids. First Lindsey, then Jake. Grateful to hear their voices. More grateful they heard mine.

CHAPTER 5
HOW DID I GET HERE

From onset of symptoms to sitting on the stretcher in the Cath Lab hallway, just shy of three hours had passed. A whirlwind of events where every decision that was made, every step, every action, every thought, so precise.

It turned out that a tiny piece of plaque, in otherwise clean arteries, erupted, blocking my right coronary artery completely. Dr. Berkery explained there is an unexpected phenomenon called plaque rupture, where there can be an inflammation inside the blood vessel wall akin to a pimple that breaks out through the skin. When that happens, the plaque will activate the clotting system, and a small 20-30% plaque blockage can progress to a 90-100% blockage in a day or two.

I imagined I might receive a stent, a tiny, expandable metal mesh coil, to keep the artery open. Instead, I received four stents— a "Full Metal Jacket"—to offer more stability due to the dissection, where the inside wall of my right coronary artery tore as the wire entered during the catheterization. A dissection is a possible risk mentioned in the consent. I sat on the stretcher smiling, chatting with the medical staff, making calls, yet fully in shock. None of this made sense to me. Nothing about this felt real, no matter how I looked at it.

The only risk factor I have is genetics. For many years I have adhered to a largely plant-based diet—no sugar, no gluten, no meat, no dairy. I am physically active, practice regular stress reduction techniques, and I neither smoke nor drink alcohol. My overall cholesterol is low with my good cholesterol high. My blood pressure is low as well and I am at a healthy body weight. At 58, I had spent the last 20 years doing everything I could to avoid this situation, yet here I was.

As I settled into my room on the Cardiac floor, my mind wandered back to when my lifestyle was a far cry from what I would call healthy. Before the last 21 years of gradually transforming how I ate, moved my body, and connected with a spiritual practice, my life looked very different. I was 275 pounds, at the tail end of an active addiction to food and compulsive overeating. A disease most people don't even know exists. It was a slow, painful path to death that I didn't know I was on, though it was the only path I knew for most of my life.

I never thought I would make it to the age of 40. Who am I kidding? I didn't think I deserved to make it to 40. How could I, knowing my mom never had the chance? When Mom died, somewhere in the back of my 13-year-old mind, I knew that I would die by 39 of a heart attack just as she did. I didn't think I had a choice, so I lived a life that supported that belief.

From my earliest memories, long before Mom died, I had an unhealthy relationship with food, always sneaking, lying, hoarding, and wanting more than everyone else. After mom died, food became both my best friend and worst enemy. As it soothed and comforted me, it also brought immense shame and guilt. The more shame and guilt I felt, the more I ate. Food, and the violent act of binging, shoved the intensity of my grief and pain deep enough that I could wake up in the morning and face the day. A day I wasn't sure I wanted to face. The thing about addiction, it doesn't let you pick and choose which emotion to quell. It suppresses them all equally.

CHAPTER 6

SETTLING INTO THE NEXT SIX DAYS

A few hours later, I sat up in the hospital bed with Lindsey beside me, seated in a chair. We were laughing and joking, and I felt perfectly fine. It seemed almost surreal that I had a heart attack—like it happened to someone else, far away. I was still on telemetry, my heart rhythm being monitored closely and transmitted to the computer screens at the nurse's station when the nurse came in with an EKG machine.

"How are you feeling?" she asked.

"I'm feeling good," I replied, expecting her to move on to the next patient.

But she didn't. She stopped at my bed, prompting me to ask, "What's up?"

"You had an 8-second run of V-tach," she explained, referring to ventricular tachycardia, which isn't uncommon after a heart attack. "We just want to take a quick look at your heart," she continued, moving closer with the EKG machine and attaching the twelve electrodes that would record my heart's rhythm and electrical signals.

Being certified in ACLS, (Advanced Cardiovascular Life Support), I knew V-tach is a serious arrhythmia where the lower chamber of the heart beats too fast to pump effectively, potentially becoming life-threatening if not corrected. I had thought I was in the clear, forgetting that the heart is not just circulatory but also electrical. I felt foolish in this oversight, and I could feel my fear rising to the surface. If my heart's electrical system went haywire, there might be no time to fix it. The realization felt like a slap in the face. A slap like in the movie *Moonstruck*, telling me to snap out of it.

The following morning, I awoke before five, as I usually do, though I wished I could've slept later after such a restless, nearly sleepless night. The IV Ativan I received at bedtime to help me sleep initially knocked me out. I was relieved to receive it via IV rather than by mouth. I was ready for the dark emptiness it would bring, and that's exactly what it did. The day quickly faded to black.

Despite the darkness the Ativan offered, I woke several times throughout the night to my roommate's frightened screams and frequent bathroom needs, each time requiring several staff members to assist her, everyone speaking in their middle-of-the-day voices, no whispers to be heard. Sleep was elusive amidst the chaos. A bit more sleep would've been nice, but I would've settled for the noise to stop.

Shortly after I woke, the CNA (certified nursing assistant) came in for my morning vital signs. Unsurprisingly, my blood pressure was 79/52. Even under the best of circumstances, it tends to run low, more like 100/68. But, with the added Metoprolol, a beta blocker usually prescribed after a heart attack to regulate heart rate, it was lower still. We had been rooting for the systolic (top) number to be over 90 since I was admitted, but no luck.

As the CNA went to report my vitals, I stared at my phone, willing time to move faster until 6:30, when I could order breakfast. I was starving. I killed time doing the daily NYT Wordle and mindlessly scrolling through social media; finally, the clock hit 6:30. I picked up the room phone and dialed the dietary extension, my mouth watering at the thought of food, though I knew it would still take 30-45 minutes to arrive.

"I'd like a bowl of oatmeal, two hard-boiled eggs, a banana, and a fresh fruit cup, please," I requested, knowing I had almonds on my nightstand for my fat.

"Would you like regular or brown sugar with that?" the voice on the other end asked.

"Neither, thank you. Just a packet of salt, please."

"I can't send up salt. You're on a cardiac diet," she replied matter-of-factly.

I was dumbfounded. A cardiac diet? I understood I had a heart attack. I wasn't in denial, but I already followed a cardiac diet in my day-to-day life. I wanted to shout, to argue that my blood pressure was low and the diet was ordered by mistake. Just send me the damn salt! But I didn't. It wasn't her fault, and she couldn't change the order. So, I just said thank you and decided to ask the nurse when she came in.

When Dr. Berkery and his entourage arrived for morning rounds, I asked about the salt. Dr. Berkery, knowing my lifestyle, looked incredulous as he asked who ordered a cardiac diet. A PA quietly admitted to it, and he instructed her to change it to a regular diet. He also promised to have the nurse bring me some salt for my oatmeal, though by then, the oatmeal was long gone, enjoyed earlier when the nurse already brought me salt. It amazes me how healthcare can so easily offer my choice of sugar but deny salt.

After 24 hours, I was given a private room. A profound relief. My first roommate had numerous needs, but the one that followed suffered from dementia and persistently asked me to help find her lost husband. As a nurse, I felt deep compassion and a strong desire to help. As a patient, uncertain of my own fate, I quietly closed the discolored, beige curtain between us and turned away. All I wanted was to be alone with my thoughts, regardless of how dull and dark they had become.

Visiting hours were restricted due to COVID. One visitor a day, from 2-6 pm. I was relieved by this limitation. It wasn't a matter of one person leaving and another arriving; it was strictly one visitor for the entire four hours. I simply didn't have the energy to talk or entertain. There was too much to process, and I craved the quiet company of my own thoughts.

My expected two-day hospital stay had stretched into six because Dr. Berkery was concerned about my EKG and echocardiogram. I had a small pericardial effusion, a buildup of fluid around the heart. Though small, it was concerning enough to require further monitoring.

Lindsey visited me daily, which was easy. We could comfortably sit in silence, talk about Chloe, be completely silly, or discuss the shock we were both still processing. The only person she would relinquish her visit for was Jake, who came to see me on Christmas. I was grateful for his presence, knowing there'd be no need for conversation or questions. We spoke maybe ten words, then settled in to watch *A Christmas Story*, which played on a two-hour loop on TV.

Some of my coworkers stopped by briefly to visit with a cup of coffee, a small Christmas present, or just to say hello, never overstaying their welcome. Others texted me regularly, asking how I was, but I often ignored them as my quiet anger grew. I couldn't answer. I didn't know how I was doing. Physically, I felt fine. Emotionally, everything was a jumble. I was grappling with feelings I'd never experienced before, emotions I couldn't even name, let alone understand enough to share. How could I explain what I didn't comprehend in a text? It felt like it was an expectation I couldn't meet, so I didn't respond. I was grateful for those who understood that a simple emoji or "thinking of you" text was enough.

CHAPTER 7

THAT WAS THEN, THIS IS NOW

I always knew that a 12-step recovery program would save my life. I'm not sure how or why, but the certainty was there. As far as I knew, there were no alcoholics in my family, so what would I know as a child about addiction and recovery? I believe it was the *ABC Afterschool Special*, "The Late Great Me: Story of a Teenage Alcoholic," that opened my eyes. When alcohol became part of my life as a teenager, I never drank alone, fearing it would make me an alcoholic. I had no idea that addiction could manifest through various substances and behaviors.

At seventeen years old, out of curiosity and happenstance, I attended my first recovery meeting, where alcohol and drug abuse were discussed. I was in a state of adolescent rebellion after my mom's death, grieving, angry, and defying authority, and it was strongly encouraged that I give it a try. I didn't see myself as an alcoholic. Yes, I drank excessively at times, blacking out and wreaking all sorts of havoc, but I also could go without it, sometimes stopping after just one or two drinks, still never drinking alone.

Sitting in that recovery meeting, surrounded mostly by the "bad boy" archetype I was drawn to, I listened to their stories. What I found fascinating was that, although I didn't think of alcohol like they shared, it was exactly how I felt about food. Little did I know then that 25 years later, I would claim my seat as an alcoholic; at that point, it was all about the food.

I was seeing a compassionate and insightful social worker at the time named Margaret. She was only six years older than I was, and for the first time since my mom died, I felt truly seen and heard. So, I decided to trust her with a secret I had never spoken aloud, my unhealthy relationship with food.

"When I sit in a recovery meeting for alcohol, I notice that I feel the same way about food as they do about alcohol," I explained quietly, avoiding eye contact. "I feel the same shame and guilt they talk about, and I relate to the idea I can't stop with just one."

I took a deep breath as I looked up into her eyes and felt her kindness as she encouraged me to go on.

"Once I take the first bite of a cookie, a French fry, a salad, whatever it is, I have to have another and another, no matter how much I beg and plead with myself to stop."

I paused, searching her face for any sign of judgment or fear. She smiled and nodded, creating a safe space for me to continue.

"It makes no sense; it doesn't matter how sternly I say to myself, *just one more*, I can't stop. The more I try, the faster, harder, and more urgently I shove it in," I confessed, still fearful of scaring her away.

"I hate my body; I hate how I feel physically, emotionally, and mentally. I hate that I will obsess over what others are eating and desperately want people to leave so I can eat in private, never letting anyone see how savagely and violently I consume food. I hate my weakness, this inability to stop. What the hell is wrong with me? It's just food!" I wondered how much I could reveal before she ran away. They all ran away when I showed too much, but she stayed, allowing me to continue.

"I've stolen food, and money to buy food. I sneak it when no one's looking, sometimes taking it from the floor, the freezer, someone's plate, and even the garbage." My heart raced as I felt sweat soaking through my shirt. She stayed, so I went on.

"I've eaten so much that my stomach hurt, then stuck my finger down my throat to get rid of it, afraid of gaining more weight, only to make room for more food," I shared, sure this would be too much for her. But it wasn't.

"I heard in a recovery meeting, 'one is too many and 100 is never enough.' That's how I feel about food, and nothing I do or say can change that," I finished, feeling a huge sense of relief. Margaret never looked away or left. There's something about shining a light on the shame that diminishes its power. She stayed and hugged me tightly. I wasn't rejected. I wasn't abandoned. This was the best purge ever, I thought as I leaned into her hug, letting myself believe in her care.

Much of my life that happened felt beyond my control, and now, with everything going on, food was at the top of the list to be addressed after sharing my deep, dark, shameful secret.

Margaret scheduled an appointment with a dietician. For the

first time in a long while, I felt hope. Maybe, just maybe, I wasn't crazy. For the first time in a long time, I didn't feel alone. I was thrilled to get some help because, as hard as it was to admit, everything until then had shown that I couldn't do it on my own.

A few days later, I sat with the dietician, enthusiastic hope tingling through my body; I blurted out, "Is there a 12-step recovery program for food like there is for alcohol?"

"That would be a good idea," she responded, "But no."

Disappointment washed over me. I had thought for sure there had to be something. Come to find out, one was founded in 1960, but we didn't know this then.

The dietician reached out, laying her hand on mine, and kindly said, "Dear, it's all about moderation."

"Moderation? Are you kidding me? If I could eat in moderation, we wouldn't be having this conversation," I retorted, rolling my eyes in annoyance.

She smiled so sweetly that I could feel the condescension oozing from her pores. "For instance," she continued, "My favorite dessert is strawberry shortcake, so I allow myself one piece every year on Fourth of July." She said this as if it were the simplest thing in the world. I sat with this for a few seconds, wondering if her ignorance was real.

"Are you fucking kidding me?" I exclaimed, mouth agape, absolutely dumbfounded. The hope that had filled me minutes earlier evaporated in a blink of an eye.

Her once-open smile tightened into a thin line. "I'll set up a plan for you," she said curtly, ending our session with a 1,000-calorie diet that I could never maintain.

Four years later, in 1985, after thumbing through the Yellow Pages, I found my way to my first 12-step recovery meeting for food at the height of my bulimia. Although I knew I belonged and understood the language they spoke, I didn't attend my second meeting until 1992, shortly after my son Brent died at three days old, born prematurely at 24.3 weeks. Again, I felt the relief of belonging, and again, I stayed away for years. Finally, in 2001, at 275 pounds and in absolute desperation, I made it to my third food recovery meeting, and there I remained, knowing I found the solution that would save my life, and was willing to stay.

Many believed I started seeking help because at 36, I was nearing 39, the age my mom died. The truth was, my daughter Lindsey was 13, and I knew with all my being I needed to do whatever I could to avoid leaving her with the same fate.

There is a saying in the group: "I came for the vanity and stayed for the sanity." For me, it was reversed. I desperately wanted the sanity. As for the vanity, I doubted I would ever eat like a so-called normal person or reach a healthy body weight. I had proven time and time again that I was incapable of sticking to any diet, and believe me, I tried them all. Cabbage soup, no sugar, no fat, no carbs, Weight Watchers, diet pills, lemon juice, purging, one meal a day, et cetera. Nothing worked. The more I tried, the more discouraged I became. The more discouraged, the more filled with self-loathing I became. The more I failed, the more I ate. A vicious cycle I couldn't escape.

Coming into the rooms of recovery was a slow process. I balked at many of the suggestions, but I was willing to show up to meetings. I had heard somewhere, "Don't leave five minutes before the miracle," and I'd be damned if the miracle showed up and I wasn't there. One day at a time, I changed how I ate. One day at a time, I worked the 12 steps, slowly incorporating them into my life. One day at a time, my perspective began to shift, as I sought to be part of the solution, not the problem. One day at a time, the weight has been released, both physically and emotionally. One day at a time, the layers of stories and lies I had protected myself with for most of my life were being peeled away. One day at a time, I am becoming the woman I am meant to be, no longer filled with shame and guilt just for existing, but with self-love, self-compassion, and self-kindness. One day at a time, I have welcomed a power greater than myself, as I understand it to be, that not only has restored me to sanity but also welcomes me into its care.

In 2006, as my son Jake approached 13, I raised the bar and gave up alcohol and began a more rigorous recovery program, one I still work to this day. Many people have questioned the disciplined nature of what I do, but if you've never experienced the soul-sucking world of addiction, it's hard to understand that this level of discipline has given me profound freedom, mind, body, and spirit.

I've been told I have amazing willpower, and I have to laugh. My so-called amazing willpower got me to 275 pounds and a life filled with chaos and pain. What I do and how I live my life today is not willpower at all. It's willingness and surrender, and I wouldn't have it any other way. My worst day today in recovery is profoundly better than my best day in active addiction.

CHAPTER 8

MOVING THROUGH
THE FOG

The six days in the hospital dragged on, each one feeling heavier than the last, as if I were sludging through quicksand. I hoped it wouldn't pull me under, yet part of me didn't care if it did. An emotion, somewhere between depression and anger, something I'd never felt before, loomed over me as if calling my name. Was it apathy? Ambivalence? Melancholy? Self-pity? Did it have a name? Did it even matter? I didn't have the energy or curiosity to try to figure it out. My mind was devoid of interesting thoughts. I had no desire to watch TV, read, or even scroll through my phone. I continued with my daily recovery writing out of sheer commitment, reading it to my sponsor each morning. But I felt like an empty shell, void of depth, purpose, or curiosity—going through the motions.

The recovery program I'm part of for food addiction requires three daily phone calls to other people in recovery. I was willing to do this; however, I kept the conversations as brief as possible, just enough to qualify as a connection. I still called my sponsor every morning, sharing my daily writing and daily inventory. The inventory involves reviewing the previous day and asking where I was resentful, selfish, dishonest, or afraid. Was I of service to others? Did I connect with my Higher Power through prayer and meditation? Do I owe anyone an apology? Et cetera...

By the fifth night, Christmas fading into the 26th, my anger came to the surface. I labeled it anger because it was easy and familiar, but if I dug a little deeper, I would see that fear and powerlessness were running the show. My mind and body felt ready to explode, and I desperately wanted to throw something—anything—and feel the satisfaction when it shattered. I had a couple of vases filled with beautiful orchids and wildflowers that had been sent to me, yet even in my rage, I couldn't bring myself to destroy them. Around two am, I jumped out of bed with a manic urgency. I ripped the sheets and pillowcases off the bed, raised them high over my head, and hurled them to the floor as hard as I could. I stood there for a moment before I began to laugh at the absurdity of it all. How utterly unsatisfying. Now, I couldn't even crawl back into bed because my sheets were crumpled on the floor. I sat in the chair, staring out into the night through the large window that spanned the entire wall, waiting for the nurse to do rounds a few hours later. I could have hit the call bell for linens sooner or even gone out in the hall to get them myself, but I felt like a toddler having a tantrum and needed to stew in my pity party a little longer.

When the nurse finally arrived, I explained what I had done, he laughed with empathy. He offered to make my bed. I thanked him but asked him to leave. I wasn't about to have him clean up my mess, and I certainly didn't want to hear any therapeutic communication that he might have offered.

By morning, I was curled in a fetal position under clean sheets when the cardiologist came in for rounds. He was a cute man, probably in his early 30s, though he looked closer to eighteen. Clearly, he'd drawn the short straw for the holiday weekend. I don't think he knew how to approach me with the palpable tension in the air.

"Good morning," he said with exaggerated cheer. "How are you this morning?"

I glared at him without blinking, "I'm angry," I growled.

"It must be hard spending Christmas in the hospital," he continued, trying to find common ground.

I stared at him incredulous. This had nothing to do with Christmas. I wanted to scream, *I am a healthy person who just had a fucking heart attack. This isn't supposed to happen to me.* Instead, I took a deep breath, locking my dark brown eyes onto his crystal blue ones, and asked, "Do you know what today is?"

He stepped back, unsure how to answer. Finally, he said, "No, I don't."

I tilted my head slightly. "It's my anniversary. I've been sober for 15 years today."

His smile softened, growing more genuine. He offered congratulations, and I smiled back, but my thoughts turned bitter. *And look where it got me.* The self-pity was suffocating as I rolled over and glared at the wall, listening to his footsteps fade as he left the room.

CHAPTER 9
MIDDLE SCHOOL REFLECTION

With endless time on my hands, my mind drifted back to an earlier memory, one where I felt just as empty and lost. It was when I first needed more than food to get through the day. It was a few months after Mom died, and while I was still trudging through thick, murky sludge, everyone else seemed to be moving forward as if nothing had happened.

Each day, I went through the motions, still unsure of where I fit in. I watched my friends and the other seventh graders, baffled by how they made life look so easy while everything felt so impossibly hard for me. I thought grief was something you went through when someone died, and then eventually, you bounced back. When Grandma, Mom's mom, died five months before Mom, I grieved. I felt the loss, the sadness, and I missed her deeply. With my family sharing stories and keeping her memory alive, it was bearable. This was different. This grief had a stranglehold on me that I couldn't shake—I didn't want to shake. It felt like if I let go of this pain, I would be letting go of her. If I let go of the anguish, It would be like saying it's okay that she's dead. And nothing about this was okay!

As I looked around at all the normalcy of life, I wanted to scream, *Don't you get it? She existed! She mattered!* How could people walk around as if she never lived? Where were her stories? I couldn't understand why no one talked about her. Eventually, I stopped talking too, stuffing everything down as far as I could—initially with food and, over time, with drugs and alcohol to numb it even further. I didn't realize it then, but all that pain, grief, and anger stuffed down eventually finds a way to spew out sideways.

I did my best to pretend I was okay, spending time with friends, hanging out at Great Games, the mall arcade, playing foosball, roller skating at Empire Skates on Friday nights. Soon enough, being the late 70s, pot became a part of the conversation. I was terrified—terrified to try it and terrified not to. It was one more way I felt like I didn't belong. I already felt awkward in my Sears Husky jeans, Dorothy Hamill haircut, and a dead mother. I was already seen as weird and different, and I would be damned if I became the butt of anyone's joke. A rebellious independence, something that had been inside me, began growing stronger, demanding to be let out, regardless of the consequences.

I spent most of my time with Judy, both in and out of school. She was the first person I smoked pot with, the first person I hitchhiked with, the first person I skipped school with, the first person I snuck out of the house with in the middle of the night. Judy was the first person I called when Mom died, months before any of that. I remember it vividly. I called her from the black rotary phone in my parents' bedroom. She answered with "Happy Easter," and I followed with, "My mom died this morning." I had been leaning against the wall, and as the words left my mouth, I felt myself slowly sinking to the floor, ending up in a seated fetal position.

We cried together, but there was nothing else to say. Judy had met my mom before, when she had come over to spend the night, however, the day before she died was the first time my mom met her mom, Mary Jane. I was at Judy's house coloring Easter eggs when Mom came to pick me up. She honked the horn of her bright yellow '75 AMC Sportabout, her first new car. I ran outside to meet her and asked her to come inside to see the eggs we colored. Of course, she did. She chatted with Mary Jane and admired our beautiful eggs. I loved sharing my mom, and Mary Jane, who had only lived in Syracuse just over a year, was happy to meet a new friend. Life was good that day. As we drove home, we chatted about all the fun I had, completely oblivious to what was to come in the next 18 hours.

CHAPTER 10

GOING HOME

After six days in the hospital, it was time to go home. Lindsey insisted I stay with her, and I was relieved to say yes. Despite my years of independence, I wasn't ready to face my little apartment alone. My movements were cautious, as if any sudden motion might push my fragile heart beyond its limits. I missed the security of the 24/7 heart monitoring. What if I didn't recognize the next time something happened?

When we arrived at Lindsey's, I sank into the soft cushions of the living room sofa, the only light coming from the Christmas tree. Its blinking lights evoked a mix of hope, love, family, and loneliness. Under the tree lay several unopened presents, with a large box of gifts yet to be placed beneath. We were waiting for the upcoming weekend to celebrate Christmas, though the word *celebrate* felt strange. Yes, I was alive, but the joy was tempered by everything I'd been through.

Having been raised Jewish, or Jew "ish," as Jake liked to call it, our Christmas traditions were always a bit inconsistent. One thing I cherished was wrapping gifts on Christmas Eve after the kids went to bed, thoughtfully placing each gift under the tree for an exciting morning surprise. This year, for the first time, I had all the gifts wrapped and stockings filled a week early as if I subconsciously knew everything needed to be ready.

After leaving the hospital Monday morning on December 27th, we decided to exchange gifts a few days later, giving me a few days to settle in. Time passed quietly. I lounged on the sofa while Lindsey, my son-in-law Keith, and 18-month-old granddaughter Chloe spent time in the family room on the other side of the house, giving me the space to process my new reality.

With me in the next room, the gate that usually closed off the family room was left open. Chloe, free to toddle out whenever she wanted, would come to the living room with a look of surprise and a big smile, exclaiming "Geeee" with delight. When Lindsey was pregnant, I found a mug that said Fairy Grandmother, and I liked the idea of being called Fairy Grandma. This evolved into "Fairy G," and that week, Chloe decided to call me "Gee," which quickly became "Gigi" by the end of my stay. My tired heart filled with joy. I loved being called Gigi and I loved this precious time with Chloe. She and I would snuggle, read books, and watch *Mickey Mouse Clubhouse* together. She couldn't quite pull herself up on the sofa, so I would lift her the last little bit, defying the doctor's orders of not to lift more than five pounds. It was our own little secret that connected me to her deeply, though Chloe ratted me out when Lindsey asked how she got on the couch. My little truthteller.

One evening, I unpacked the big box of gifts that Lindsey had brought from my apartment, placing them under the tree and setting out the already-filled stockings. I let the love I felt fill me up. A few days later, Jake came over, and we exchanged gifts. We laughed and enjoyed Chloe's wonder and excitement as she passed out our presents and helped us open them.

On the first Monday of 2022, Lindsey brought me to my apartment. A new year. A new life. She tried to convince me to stay at her house for one more week. I considered it, but ultimately, I wanted to go home. I could easily have stayed curled up on her sofa for several more days, but I needed to return to the scene of the crime, so to speak, and start moving forward. I managed to slowly climb up the 15 steep wooden stairs that I was carried down only 13 days earlier. The fear of overexerting my heart weighed heavily on me. Lindsey had shoveled the steps a few days earlier, making it safe to ascend, but after Chloe and I walked into my living room, Lindsey went out to shovel the steps again.

Chloe went to the cupboard where I keep her books, and I stood staring at the round, fluffy, purple rug in the middle of the room where I had knelt down and called 911. The thoughts from that Solstice morning rushed back, disbelief washing over me once again. Did I really have a heart attack and almost die? It still made no sense.

Lindsey brought the rest of my things up and sat down in the other multicolored floral chair next to mine. We made small talk, avoiding the heaviness of the moment.

"Are you sure you don't want to come back to my house for a few more days," Lindsey asked, her tone to make it light, with a little laugh.

"I'd love to, honey, but I need to be here," I replied.

"I know. I thought I'd try one more time," she said with a playful smile.

We hugged tightly before she gathered up Chloe to leave. I hugged them both, and we simultaneously said, "I love you."

I closed the door behind them, turning the deadbolt as it shut. I leaned my back against the door and looked around the kitchen. Everything was exquisitely quiet. I could feel it at a cellular level, the silence moving slowly through my body, a stark contrast to the frantic movements of that fateful morning. Here I was, now standing in the future that had once been so uncertain. Now what?

I walked into the small living room, noticing that everything was exactly how I left it. The round purple rug in the middle of the room, the large plants filling a quarter of the space, the two wildly-flowered chairs at one end, even the sun shining through the windows—it was all the same. I sat in one of the chairs. The chair I always chose. The chair where it all began.

CHAPTER 11
EARLY CONTEMPLATION

As I sat there, I was filled with contradictions that defied logic. I was deeply alone, yet not lonely. My emotions surged within me, yet I was numb. I had a keen awareness of thoughts, yet I couldn't find meaning in them. I was physically in the room, yet mentally somewhere else. It felt like I was experiencing trauma. Was it post-traumatic, or was I still in the midst of it?

I have experienced significant traumas in my life, traumas that were undeniable, but this, was this considered a trauma? What qualifies as trauma, I wondered?

My mother's death when I was thirteen was a trauma. The loss of my son Brent, born at 24.3 weeks, dying 72 hours later, was a trauma. Years of emotional abuse, gaslighting, and rape were traumas. Living in addiction and all that entails was a trauma. Being institutionalized in my late teens, begging to be heard, was a trauma. But this? This was an event. It was quick. Treatable. Death was a possibility, but I never felt it calling me. Yes, I felt powerless, even though I knew what to do, who to call, where to go. Trauma? Really?

As I wrestled with what I was feeling, more so in my head with thoughts than feelings in my body, I considered the possibility that this could be an acute trauma. A sudden, unforeseen, and distressing experience that can lead to anxiety, grief, shock, sadness, and denial. I wondered, my mom's death was a sudden, unexpected, stressful event, yet over time, it became what I would call chronic trauma, arising from repeated exposure to stress and grief. Although she didn't die over and over again, my response to her death led to choices and situations no adolescent should have to endure repeatedly. Maybe it was more complex trauma, where acute and chronic merge.

I wanted to scream, overwhelmed by it all. What was the point of figuring this out? Did any of it even matter? The weight of it felt too much to bear, so I decided to shelve the thoughts for another day.

I shut my eyes, trying to meditate, but that, too, felt overwhelming. I stood up and began pacing my 450-square-foot apartment, searching for something to do. Whether by synchronicity, coincidence, or divine intervention, there was nothing to be done. When I left the apartment thirteen days ago, the dishes were washed and put away, my clothes surprisingly folded and out of sight. Even the garbage had been taken out two hours before I left in the ambulance. Only my bed remained unmade, and I didn't have the energy to make it. This was not typical of how I live. I wish it were. I wish I were tidier and more organized—but I'm not. Yet, there I was, in awe of how I left my apartment. I choose to believe the universe knew what I was about to face and prepared me for it. After all, I'd even had all the Christmas gifts and stockings filled, ready to go in a big box.

CHAPTER 12
FIRST FOLLOW-UP APPOINTMENT

The next day, I arrived for my two-week follow-up, expecting to see Dr. Berkery. Instead, I was surprised and immediately disheartened to find that my appointment was with his PA, Riley. I had never met her before, and a wave of disappointment, anger, and even betrayal washed over me. I wanted Dr. Berkery. I needed him. He knew me, my heart, my history.

Riley began to speak, her tone and words different from Dr. Berkery's in the hospital. My body tensed. My fists clenched in my lap as my shoulders crept toward my ears. Her words became a blur, a distant buzz, like the adults in a Peanuts cartoon, *Wah wa wah* was all I could hear.

"I'm sure you're very good at your job, but I need to see Dr. Berkery," I blurted out, surprising myself with the harshness of my tone. I couldn't go along with this for one more second.

"He's here if you'd like me to go get him," she said calmly.

"Yes, please," I managed to say, barely containing my agitation.

A few minutes later, Dr. Berkery entered the room, with Riley trailing behind him. Relief flooded my body. I exhaled a breath I didn't realize I'd been holding. My fists unclenched and my shoulders relaxed. The only tension left was in my eyes as I fought to hold back tears.

"Tell me about your anger," Dr. Berkery encouraged without preamble, his gaze steady. There was no small talk, no pretense. Just, "Tell me about your anger," meeting me exactly where I was.

"I am so fucking angry," I admitted, finally acknowledging the depth of my rage.

"I'm angry that I had a heart attack after years of doing everything I could to avoid it. I am angry that I have to take three new prescriptions, a blood thinner, something for cholesterol, and a beta blocker to keep my heart rate low, when I don't want to take any. I am angry that I now have to add coronary artery disease to my health history," I said, my voice controlled but seething. I took a deep breath before continuing, "And I am so fucking angry that I am powerless over my body."

He held the space in silence, allowing me to finish, ensuring I had said all that needed to be said.

He reassured me that what I was feeling was normal. I had heard that anger and depression were common after a heart attack but to experience it was something else entirely. Ironically, knowing it was normal only made me angrier and more depressed.

Dr. Berkery reviewed the follow-up plan with me. I would see him again at six weeks, six months, and then a year, with the door open if I had any concerns in between. I liked having a plan. It provided some relief from the uncertainty, despite not giving me the answers I craved. He cleared me to return to work in a week. Physically, I knew three weeks would be sufficient. I only worked two ten-hour shifts a week with occasional on-call thrown in. But emotionally, it felt too soon. I was still processing what had happened, what was happening, what would happen. I wasn't ready.

Sensing my hesitation, he added another week, giving me a full month before returning to work, offering me longer if I needed. One month felt doable, and I agreed.

CHAPTER 13

MEETING MY ANGER AND WHAT LURKS BENEATH

The following week, I spent a great deal of my time sitting in my chair. The ever present funkily colored floral chair that had become my touchstone. This was the chair that I felt the first twinge of a heart attack. It's the chair where I think, reflect, talk on the phone, meditate, eat my meals, watch TV, write, and process my life. Over two years later, it is the chair I am sitting in as I write these words.

I picked up my copy of Brene Brown's *Atlas of the Heart*, hoping to better understand what I was feeling. As I read her definition of anger, I was reminded that anger can be an umbrella, covering a variety of other emotions beneath it. Emotions that may be harder to name and even harder to feel. I felt anger but not angry, and this made no sense to me, so in my typical fashion, I knew I needed to look under the canopy and explore a little deeper.

I've always been an emotional digger, driven by an insatiable desire to better understand myself at the deepest level. I opened my laptop and pulled up an old piece I wrote in 2016 while spending a month in Peru:

Spending so much time in the desert, I realized that I have always considered myself a digger... An archeologist of the self. I set out to lost lands to discover answers, the truth, authenticity ... pieces of me that I have lost along the way. I am willing to do the hard work and I dig, and I dig until, alas, I find a treasure. It may be an awareness, an "aha" moment, a realization of a deeper sense of who I am. I hold it up with a smile and a sense of accomplishment, and I shout, "EUREKA ... look at this beautiful treasure that I have found." I then toss it aside into an ever-growing pile of the many other neglected riches that I have exposed over the years and start digging for the next. Oh, the many treasures that I have discarded, excited for the find, yet not taking the time to polish its beauty to make it shine, not pausing to brush out the crevices to allow for the essence of each treasure to expand and express its true self. How sad to dig for the next without honoring the prior. Today, I will take out my excavation tools, and I will rub and buff each gem, one at a time. I will clean out every nook and cranny, casting away any fear of what I may find embedded into these deep openings. It is time to allow the excess layers to peel away, and with complete vulnerability and transparency, I will stand naked in my truth, living fully in the I AM...

These words were what I needed to read. What is this anger trying to tell me? If I don't take the time to truly examine it, to brush away the debris, and listen deeply, it will swallow me whole. I am not an angry person by nature. Sure, I've experienced anger, a state of being, a moment in time, a reaction to an event, not a defining trait. So, to carry this weight around my neck, pulling me down, made me afraid that this was becoming my new normal. And I couldn't accept that. I wouldn't accept that.

In the quiet of the room, I reminded myself that anger wasn't the only thing I had been feeling. I also experienced gratitude, hope, and joy. It's funny—I never question why I feel hopeful, grateful, or happy. I don't stop in the middle of a joyful moment to ask, *Why me?* I don't interrupt my laughter to analyze it. I just laugh. I'm just happy. I'm just grateful. But the darker, heavier feelings, such as anger, grief, sadness, and depression, those I feel compelled to explore. I wonder though, by seeking their purpose, am I avoiding feeling them as deeply?

Seeking has its place in my growth and healing. Over the years, it has opened up my mind, eyes, and heart. It has shifted my perception of people, events, and experiences in profoundly positive ways. *And*, seeking has also been a tool I have subconsciously used to avoid feelings, outcomes, and the truth. The magical thinking that if I can just figure it out, then I can take action and fix it. In hindsight, I realize this is just another avoidance technique. The truth is, most things don't need to be figured out or fixed. They just need to be accepted, experienced, and integrated—moving through, moving on, or moving with.

Despite this awareness, in that moment, I needed to seek. I needed to meet this emotion where it was. Sitting in the same chair that always supports me, I decided to face this bully called anger head-on. I pulled out my notebook, and at the top of the page, I wrote, "This is your anger, and this is what I want you to know." This is a tool I have used many times—giving voice to an emotion, a thought, an idea that I can't quite reach with my own self-knowledge. It allows me to tap into my intuition, my higher self, if I can just get out of the way and let it speak.

Dear Caron,

This is your anger, and this is what I want you to know. You are playing the role of the victim. You are feeling wronged, as if you are being punished unfairly, and I am here to tell you, that's bullshit. I, as your anger, am an easy scapegoat. It's familiar, understandable and it makes sense. You internally whine that this wasn't supposed to happen to you. You point out to yourself that you have gone to great lengths to live a healthy lifestyle. You have done everything right, and still, here you are. It's as if you are standing on a mountaintop in a superhero pose. Standing straight, shoulders back, chin out, fisted hands to your hips, legs squared beneath you. There is a self-righteousness, growling, "Don't you know who I am?" As if because of the work you have done in your healing journey, you are above this physical weakness. Yes, you see it as a weakness. Peel back the anger and look more deeply. Is that shame that you see? Shame in not just a physical weakness, but you see it also as a moral weakness. A childish belief that you should know better, do better, be better. You see the arrogance in that, don't you?

I paused in the writing, rereading what I had just written. I put my head in my hands as the words sank in, feeling their truth.

Seeing the shame and arrogance in their totality. How ridiculous, I thought. Who did I think I was to be exempt from life on life's terms? Embarrassment washed over me. Or was it humility? At that moment, I was unsure.

CHAPTER 14

MY RELATIONSHIP WITH WRITING

I leaned back in the chair, closing my eyes as I remembered the day I was introduced to the saving grace of writing. I had always enjoyed telling a story, embellishing real-life situations to make them more exciting or interesting. If it was a mile, I made it three. If there were snowflakes, I turned them into a blizzard. Exaggeration, dramatization, even lying—these came naturally to me, so much so that I would often forget what was true and what I created. This habit colored my verbal storytelling, but when it came to writing, that's where I found the truth.

When Mom died, I wanted to express my feelings, despite not knowing the words to name them. Words like grief and sadness felt too general, too small to describe the depth and intensity of what I was experiencing. Years later, I learned it was anguish and despair that I had felt. At the time, as much as I wanted to, talking about my emotions was challenging. It quickly became clear that my feelings made people uncomfortable. Throughout my childhood, I had always sensed that my energy was too much for those around me. During that time of loss and rebellion, I realized it wasn't just me that was too much, it was also my feelings. People would avoid me, change the subject, or worse, they'd cry. The pity I would see in their eyes was constant. I hated being pitied. It made me feel weak and inferior, compounding the overwhelming sense of rejection and abandonment I was already grappling with.

I was only thirteen. My grandmother died at 61 after years of battling a debilitating disease called Shy-Drager Syndrome, (think Parkinson's on crack). Five months later, my mother suddenly died at 39 of a heart attack. Eleven days after that, our ten-year-old dog, Timmy, died—from what we were told, a broken heart. Of course, people ran away from me. This was too much for anyone. I was too much for anyone. In my traumatized adolescent mind, I couldn't distinguish between the experiences happening and my identity. To me, they were one and the same.

I was placed in therapy with the only child psychologist in our area in the late 1970s. Although I was thrilled to finally have someone to share my thoughts and feelings with, someone who could help me dig deeper into who I was, I didn't trust her. At thirteen, I had no understanding of energy or why I was repelled by certain people, but I knew enough to recognize when I was attracted and when I was repelled. And I was repelled by her. However, she did encourage me to journal and that suggestion I took to heart.

I grabbed a spiral notebook and a pen, starting with a few tentative words, like dipping my toe into the ocean to test the temperature and the strength of the waves. Slowly, over time, I waded up to my knees, words flowing easier and with more meaning. Finally, with great excitement, wonder, and anticipation, I dove in head-first, letting the giant wave take me under, wrapping me in the safety of its eye.

There was an urgency and insistence to my writing. It became my life raft, my oxygen tank, it kept me afloat, allowing me to breathe again. It was the only place where the truth of what I was feeling and who I was could find its way to the surface. For the next five years, I carried a notebook and a thesaurus with me everywhere. I would stop whatever I was doing, wherever I was—at the mall, a friend's house, at school—and write whenever something needed to come out. It was in my writing, whether journaling, poetry, or short stories, that I formed a relationship with my grief, connecting me with my mom through my expression. It was in my writing that the truth, *my* truth, was safe. I could tell my story without embellishment or lies. Though my feelings were always big, and often dramatic, the pages of my notebooks could handle it. I was never too much for them. If it weren't for my writing and the safety that it offered to express everything within me, I believe I would've died. I have no doubt that writing saved my life.

At eighteen, I stopped writing abruptly, with a tremendous amount of sadness. An acquaintance had found one of my poems and published it in a small community magazine under her name. I felt profoundly violated and betrayed. The safety I once felt was shattered, and I couldn't write with any truth again until I was 43 years old, when writing became a requirement of my recovery. Despite the requirement, I was hesitant to dive too deeply. The sting of that earlier betrayal remained, compounded by another when I was 21—an ex-boyfriend stole and burned my notebooks filled with poetry, grief, my words of connection with my mom, my hopes, dreams, and fears. Those notebooks held *ME*. They contained the truth of who I was—who I am. I was devastated. I still grieve the loss of those words written so long ago.

Slowly, over time, my trust in the words and those I shared them with returned, breaking down the wall I had built, allowing my truth to resurface. Though I have yet to write another poem, I have not missed a day of writing in the last seventeen years. Always my recovery writing, often my morning pages as taught in Julia Cameron's *The Artist's Way,* and the on-again, off-again relationship with my memoir. Writing is no longer a necessity for me to breathe; it remains a necessity for my ongoing healing. It allows me to find the truth in what I'm thinking and feeling when I can't see it clearly on my own.

CHAPTER 15

BACK TO ANGER

I opened my eyes to find myself sitting in my chair, staring at the letter I had been writing from anger. I paused, said a quick prayer, and asked the universe what else needed to be said. Taking a deep breath, I continued, letting the anger guide my words, hoping it would reveal what I needed to know.

The voice on the page continued.

I can see you acknowledge your shame and arrogance. Like anger, they are emotions that prevent you from telling the full story. Yes, they play a role, making you feel as if you have some control, but there are deeper layers that scare the shit out of you. I want to take you deeper into the truth, down to the place that makes you squirm with discomfort. The place that makes you want to run and hide. The place you want to deny because you are strong and resilient and if you go there you feel weak and incompetent. A little secret before I take you to this place. Please know, it is a lie. You are not weak and incompetent. Not when it comes to this. Not ever.

The place I want to show you is betrayal. I can see you flinch simply with the written word. Betrayal is a deep violation– a violation of trust. Trust in another person; trust in yourself. Can you see the truth in this? Can you feel the validity?

Shame, anger, arrogance, betrayal. They are all valid. There is no limit to the emotions that may arise from this experience. You've never faced anything like this before, so whatever comes up is uncharted territory. I ask you not to judge yourself or your emotions. Allow whatever wants to be heard, be heard. Give yourself permission that whatever wants to be felt, be felt. They are not your enemies, they are your guides.

With encouragement and faith, you will find your way,

Anger

I reread all that was written, feeling the storm they stirred within me. Of all the emotions, exhaustion rose to the top. This felt like too much, but I couldn't turn away. Why did this hurt so much? What was this betrayal, and how did it affect me? Just the word *betrayal* twisted something deep beneath my skin, and I couldn't shake it loose. This was the kind of discomfort I once buried under excessive food and alcohol, but not today. Today, I choose to face my feelings, to understand them, and allow them their voice no matter how uncomfortable it makes me. I can't get to the truth if I'm not willing to bushwhack my way through the weeds, and these hard emotions are my thicket.

CHAPTER 16

COMING TO TERMS WITH BETRAYAL

I thought back to when I first felt betrayal and what it triggered within me. It wasn't hard to pinpoint. Doesn't all the hard stuff go back to Mom's death? I know I was *me* the thirteen years before she died, but like it is for so many, there's that one event that splits our lives in two. A before and an after. And so much of who I am today is rooted in the after. It shaped me in ways that nothing else could have.

Betrayal is a violation of trust, and after Mom died, everything I trusted disappeared. It wasn't just losing Mom and our dog Timmy; I lost the father I always knew and relied on. First to his grief and then, when he remarried 18 months later, to his new wife. I lost my sister, who went off to college, rarely coming home, as she dealt with her own feelings in her own way, 150 miles away. I lost my aunts, Mom's two sisters, and my cousins who lived two hours away, still gathering with each other but seldom including me. I lost the home I grew up in when Dad and his new wife sold it and moved us to the neighborhood where my mom had always wanted to live. At 13, I lost my childhood, leaving it behind as I attempted to forge my way into this new, foreign, and lonely territory.

I knew intellectually that it was not Mom's fault. That she would never have chosen to leave. She didn't intentionally betray me. It took me many years, therapy, and a variety of other healing modalities to acknowledge, understand, and resolve the betrayal I felt from her death but couldn't name. At 13, I trusted her more than anyone in this world, and she left me. No goodbye. No explanation. Just gone. But at the time, I refused to blame her or be angry with her. I refused to betray her. While everyone else seemed to be moving on with their lives, I remained loyal. I held onto her the only way I knew how, with the intensity of my grief that I gripped with the tenacity of an angry dog protecting its bone, growling and baring my teeth at anyone who came near, while simultaneously longing to be rescued.

At 58, my grief was still with me, yet we had transformed our relationship. We had learned to live in harmony together, dancing and breathing, with an occasional necessary hiccup of tears and longing. Now, reading the words I had just written from my anger, I asked myself: What did betrayal mean today? What trust was violated?

The word "powerless" comes to mind. My body betrayed me, despite how well I treated it for the past 15-plus years. I did the work, trusting my body to carry me through, believing we were on the same team, convinced it had my back. I knew I wasn't immortal, but I never thought my heart would betray me after all the love I had given it.

Over the years in recovery, I have come to terms with the reality that I am powerless over food and alcohol. When I don't accept that, my life quickly becomes unmanageable. That's step one of the 12 steps in recovery. Yet somehow, I fooled myself into thinking I had control over my body. How naive. I'm a nurse; I spent years working in organ donation. I witnessed healthy people succumbing to sudden death despite how well they lived their lives time and time again. Why did I ... How did I think I was any different? Any better?

This realization triggered something in me I thought was healed. I felt a sense of self-betrayal as well, feeling naïve, gullible, and a bit foolish. For years, one of my greatest fears was to look stupid, appearing as if I wasn't in the know. I was terrified of being taken advantage of, so I thought I always needed to be one step ahead. But, with all the healing I have done—physically, emotionally, intellectually, and spiritually—I have learned to laugh at myself when I mess up. I have learned the well-earned lesson of being teachable and being able to say, *I don't know.* This has empowered me with self-love and self-compassion. It has allowed me to be comfortable in my skin. And still, here I was, thinking I could've, should've done more.

The truth I felt in reading this letter cracked me open just enough to remind me that my emotions are not my identity. They are visitors at this moment, and they will not overstay their welcome if I shine a light on them instead of burying them in denial. My feelings will not kill me, but they can maim me, paralyze me, if I don't acknowledge them and hear what they need to say. I can then offer a quick thank you and ask them to be on their way.

Tears slowly found their way down my cheeks as I acknowledged that I did the best I could. None of this was my fault, just as Mom's death wasn't hers. I missed her so much as I felt the fullness of humility. I am human. She was human. It is a tenuous path we humans walk each day, never truly knowing when or how it will end.

CHAPTER 17
BACK TO WORK

J anuary 18, 2022. I could hardly believe four weeks had passed, and here I was heading back to the PACU (Post-Anesthesia Care Unit) at Crouse Hospital for a 10-hour shift. *Would any of this ever make sense to me?* I wondered. Despite the uncertainty, I found myself looking forward to returning to work. It was gratifying to see my coworkers, as well as having something to do with my time and being of service. I can enjoy my own company, but that past month, I had grown weary of myself. A dullness had settled in, and I was eager to squeegee it away, like clearing the dead bugs off my windshield after a long road trip.

I was welcomed back with great big bear hugs and a barrage of well-meaning, if somewhat jarring, comments that seemed to both comfort and validate my feelings of failure, embarrassment, and betrayal.

"If this can happen to you, what hope do we have?"

"This is why I don't live a healthy lifestyle!"

"All that healthy eating and still look what happens!"

"I can't believe this happened to you, of all people!"

And on it went, everyone wanting to hear all the details. I found myself retelling the story over and over as colleagues, hearing about my ordeal for the first time, asked about my symptoms, what finally made me call 911, shocked that I lied to the 911 operator.

I was grateful I had the extra week off before my return to work because a week ago, this would've been too much to handle emotionally. But now, I was ready to share it in small doses. What surprised me most was how many healthcare professionals were unaware that women present differently than men when having a heart attack. Their shock at this revelation was almost as shocking to me as the event itself. How was this not common knowledge?

At that moment, I knew that somehow, someday, I would need to shout this fact from the rooftops. I felt a strong urge to educate the masses, though I knew I had a great deal of healing to do before I could even begin to figure out how to do this or what it would look like. In many ways, I felt like a baby deer, struggling to steady my wobbly legs beneath me. But I also knew that as I grew stronger—physically, emotionally, and mentally—it would be my responsibility to share this knowledge.

CHAPTER 18

SECOND FOLLOW-UP APPOINTMENT

In early February, I attended my six-week follow-up appointment with Dr. Berkery. He was pleased with how well I was doing. The echocardiogram showed that my heart was healing well, though it was still a bit sludgy, likely due to the dissection and stents. Dr. Berkery assured me that this was expected and the healing will continue.

"My anger seems to have lessened, but what about this dullness I'm experiencing?" I asked.

"Tell me more about it," He urged.

"Is it depression? Fear? I don't know." I replied, pausing as I tried to find the right words.

"It's not that I'm bored; it's more like apathy, a monotonous droning in what feels like an empty head. I've heard depression is common after a heart attack but for how long?" And then, with curiosity, I asked, "How do I even know this is depression? I don't feel what I would describe as melancholy or sadness."

"It's different for everyone," he said, his tone apologetic, as if he wished he could solve this puzzle for me.

"I know exercise can help with depression," I continued, "But I'm afraid to exert my heart. I'm constantly watching my Fitbit, and when my heart rate goes over 100, I stop whatever I'm doing and focus on my breathing to slow it down."

"I want your heart rate to go up and stay up," he encouraged. "Get it up to 120, 140 even, and keep it there for 20-30 minutes. Your heart can handle it," he reassured me.

Like so many things in my life, I believed it was true for others but doubted it for myself, as if I was terminally unique. That I was somehow the exception. I wanted to believe him—I truly did—but I was scared. A little over a month ago, I had a perfect echocardiogram, so I didn't know what to trust. What if my increased heart rate triggered an arrhythmia, and this time, I didn't have time to get help? This wasn't supposed to happen to me in the first place. How could I be sure it wouldn't happen again? He listened, he encouraged, he supported but he couldn't guarantee.

We talked about travel, as I had plans to fly to Nashville, Tennessee, to visit my friend Gwen the following week and fly again to Charlotte, North Carolina, in April to visit my friend Julie. Was it safe to fly? Could the air pressure in the plane be harmful? What if I had another heart attack while I was in the air? What if, what if, what if? I didn't like this new anxious side of me. This wasn't how I lived my life. I used to love to travel and enjoyed flying. This overthinking was exhausting. Dr. Berkery assured me it was safe to travel and was pleased I had plans. I decided to believe him.

Six weeks earlier, I had chosen to live and called 911. Now, I faced the challenge of truly living this life. The phrase, "You only live once," came to mind, but I was reminded that the truth is, you only die once—you live every day. I had often heard that people who have near-death experiences emerge with a renewed zest for life, eager to take big bites out of it, recognizing its fragility and seizing every moment. Was my heart attack truly a near-death experience if I never felt a sense of impending doom? As I wondered when this dullness would pass, I also wondered how I would show up for my life when it did.

CHAPTER 19

NASHVILLE

As I sat on the plane, preparing to take off to Nashville, a wave of guilt washed over me, settling behind my eyes. When Gwen and I made the plans for my visit, I was so excited. Now, though, I didn't want to go. A few days earlier, I had even called Gwen to tell her I couldn't make it. It all felt too much. Not only was I recovering from a heart attack, but this was also my first flight since COVID and all the accompanying concerns. On top of that, Gwen had made all sorts of plans for us. This was a major difference between us: she found comfort in plans, while I preferred to let the day unfold naturally. I amusingly call this *planned spontaneity*. I had to nix the Super Bowl party where I would meet her friends and the live music event she had arranged the evening I arrived. I felt incredibly selfish saying no to her efforts to share her life in Nashville, but I couldn't bring myself to say a codependent "yes" just to make her happy. It would've led to resentment, and for me, guilt was a safer emotion to process. Resentment could cause me to say or do something I'd regret. Lately, I had become inexplicably exhausted, both physically and emotionally, and making plans felt more than I could handle.

I love spending time with Gwen. She brings out a side of me that feels truly alive. She is my adventure buddy. In 2015, we spent ten days in Costa Rica together, ziplining across the lush green canopy of Monteverde, whitewater rafting through the Class 3 rapids of the Tenorio River, rappelling down the waterfalls in a remote village in the middle of the jungle, and parasailing after a brief lesson, all in Spanish, which looked like a game of charades. Neither of us spoke Spanish well, and we held on for dear life as the boat lifted us up into the air.

Gwen is my hiking companion—she, the proficient, prepared expert; me the novice, far less prepared but always eager for the adventure. It was Gwen who was with me when I broke my ankle in the High Peaks of the Adirondacks. We were descending, basking in the glow of achievement after summiting two of the 46 High Peaks, Phelps and Tabletop. She stayed by my side, encouraging me and making me laugh as I was carried miles down the mountain in a litter by four strangers, one of whom was a hyper woman eating chocolate-covered coffee beans like popcorn. The journey, lit only by our headlamps, continued long after the sun had set.

It was Gwen I was with, hiking a portion of the Appalachian Trail in East Tennessee, when we were caught in a sudden torrential downpour. With no trees or caves to offer shelter, just wide-open terrain, we were exposed to the full force of the storm. Gwen, of course, had prepared for bad weather; I, in just a tank top, shorts, and hiking boots, had hoped for the best. We moved as quickly as we could to the lot, where her car waited patiently for our arrival.

Step after step, we sang, told stories, and laughed, trekking through the rain and hoping to see the car around the next bend. As my mind grew foggy, my steps became unsteady, and my words less coherent, Gwen recognized the early signs of hypothermia, and with nowhere to hide from the storm, she got us to the car.

Gwen, my fellow emotional digger—no topic off limits. We discuss God, spirituality, fears, dreams, addiction, recovery, family, love, therapy, relationships, emotions, ideas, goals, resistance, procrastination, success, and failure. We can talk for hours, offering feedback, therapizing, sharing secrets, calling each other out on our bullshit, and telling hard truths. Everything is welcome to the table. It is safe and encouraged to be our authentic selves, with deep love and respect.

As the airplane took off, I closed my eyes and said the Serenity Prayer, as I always do when I fly: "God grant me the serenity to accept the things I cannot change, the courage to change the things I can, and the wisdom to know the difference."

After the brief feeling of peace from the prayer, the guilt returned. So much for the serenity prayer, I thought with a laugh. All I could think of was disappointing Gwen. Despite my telling her that all I wanted was to spend time with her, I knew she was likely planning activities to ensure I had the best experience possible.

Physically I was scared to do much—definitely no hiking, maybe a walk. Emotionally, my mind was void of depth, wallowing in dullness. Spiritually, I wouldn't say I was faithless, yet I felt somewhat disconnected. I knew Gwen would eventually honor my needs, but for the first time in our 21-year friendship, our 16-year age difference, me 58, she 42, I felt old.

I arrived at 11:30 am and took an Uber to her apartment, giving me more time alone with my thoughts, searching for anything positive. Gwen arrived home after work at 3:30, and with our giant octopus-like hug, wrapping our limbs around each other, the negativity lifted.

Over the next few days, we shared so much laughter and companionship. She eased off trying to make plans. We took a few simple walks, and I met a few of her friends, sharing stories of our lives, laughter deep from the belly, tears streaming down our faces. I didn't confide all the fears and darkness I was feeling because, to be honest, I didn't know how to verbalize it. I was still processing. Gwen is usually a friend I would turn to for that, but this seemed like something I had to navigate on my own.

After so many years of friendship, with big activities and adventure off the table, we found ourselves needing to connect in new ways. We finally decided to curl up on the couch, snuggling comfortably in the physical affection of our friendship, and binged the fourth season of *Yellowstone*, which, as it turned out, was exactly what we both needed.

As we discovered new ways to show our love, care, and consideration for each other, I was reminded of my dad and the many times we had to find new footing in our relationship. My dad was not known for his ability to communicate. He could get angry quickly but didn't know how to express it well, nor did he have any desire to explore what lay beneath his anger. He also loved deeply, but that, too, was often murky and unclear. His one consistent expression of love was through his cooking and baking. He excelled at both and shared his culinary creations generously.

As I grew in my recovery, my dietary choices changed. First removing sugar and gluten, then gradually eliminating meat and dairy. Dad tried to accommodate my needs, which, to me, showed his love more than any meal ever could. But it frustrated him. Eventually, it became easier for me to bring my own food. I remember the moment that we agreed to do things differently. Once again he tried to create a meal I could eat, and once again, there was something in it I didn't eat. I looked at him with so much love and said, "Dad, thank you so much for trying, but I think it's time you find a new way to show you love me." He kissed me on the side of my head and never tried again with the food. In that moment, something shifted within both of us. There was an acceptance and love for each other, along with the willingness to allow the other to be who we are—at least where it came to food—without another word needing to be spoken.

Spending time with Gwen and recalling this moment with my dad made me realize I was in a new place, a new season, where I needed to renegotiate with myself. What do I want? How am I showing up? What is it I need to do? What am I willing to do? At that moment, I had no idea.

CHAPTER 20

TRYING TO GET TO PAM

Time dragged on, and I did my best to smile and laugh, pretending all was well. I'm not sure who I was pretending for—my friends, my family, my coworkers, myself? I knew I should be grateful, and in many ways, I was, but behind closed doors, it was hard to live as if that were true. I found it increasingly difficult to know what I believed or where I belonged. The one thing I knew for sure was I had to lean close to my recovery, using the tools that had carried me through life's challenges before. So, I continued my daily practices of weighing and measuring my food, calling my sponsor, taking my sponsee's calls each morning, making my three outreach calls to others in recovery, and doing my reading and writing assignment using recovery literature. If nothing else, I could do this. It kept me connected to my Higher Power, and that faith was the lifeline I needed to get through each day.

My next trip was approaching, one I had preplanned prior to my cardiac event. This time, I was hesitant to go, but for completely different reasons. My cousin Pam, Aunt Marge's daughter, two years younger than me, was dying of cancer 300 miles away in Virginia. Pam and I had been so close as children despite the two-hour drive between Syracuse and Albany. Our families made the trip often, and we saw each other regularly. When mom died, we saw each other less and less. Long-distance rates were too expensive, and without social media or texting in the 70s and 80s, we were left to the actions, or inactions, of the adults around us. Years passed with little interaction. Even when Pam attended Syracuse University for four years, we saw each other only a few times. Adolescence had changed us both, and we didn't know how to meet each other where we were. But our love remained strong.

As adults with families of our own, neither of us initiated much connection. My children were much older than hers, and we only saw each other at the occasional family reunion or random event. Each time, it was wonderful to see her, and we'd laugh, reminisce, and get to know each other's families a little more. We'd make promises to get together, with the truest of intentions, but we never followed through. Still, whenever we did meet, it was like falling in love with each other all over again.

After seven years of living with and without cancer, Pam was out of time. Hospice was involved, and her days on Earth were coming to a close. I asked to visit, and I was told no. Pam didn't want anyone there. I wanted to beg and plead, to remind them who I was. The twelve-year-old in me wanted to kick and scream, to shout that I was part of the family and deserved to be let in. The adult in me wanted to point out that I am a nurse, trained and certified in end-of-life care and grief coaching. This was where I shined. I could help. No matter how I approached them, my offer was declined. I understood this was about Pam, not me, but it still hurt.

All the rejection and abandonment I felt when Mom died came rushing back. I had to pull out every tool I had in my toolbox to stay grounded in what I knew to be true. In end-of-life care, it is about respecting the wishes of the person who is dying. It's their experience, and I honor that deeply.

Despite that knowledge, I let my emotions drive the decision to make the 300-mile trip to see her. I told myself that I'd just give her a quick hug and turn around and go home. I rationalized that once they saw me, they'd remember that I belonged there and would invite me in. I longed for that acceptance, not just in this moment but throughout my life. I ignored the inner voice reminding me how selfish I was being. Feeling, for the first time since the heart attack, a sense of urgency and purpose, I got in the car. Helping people transition into death and supporting their families through grief is a gift I have. A calling aligned with my reason for still being alive. I took a deep breath, started the car, and I said a prayer. "Please, Dear Universe, guide me on this journey. If this is the right decision, may I travel with ease. If not make it so clear to me I can't deny it—sooner rather than later."

An hour out of Syracuse, heading down I-81 South, I hit a pothole I didn't see. The undercarriage of my car dropped. I pulled over and managed to rig it enough to stay up. I knew it was safer to head back home than continue to Virginia. I turned the car around, back onto I-81 North, and drove home, recognizing that my prayer was answered, even if it wasn't the outcome I wanted.

CHAPTER 21

NORTH CAROLINA

Not feeling needed or welcomed by my family, I found myself back on an airplane, this time heading to Charlotte, North Carolina, to visit Julie. It was a trip I'd either flown or driven every year for the last nine years, since her husband, Jim, died. Julie and I had been friends since we were fifteen. She moved to Syracuse to live with her father, and we bonded over our love of partying, Janis Joplin, and a mutual disdain for our stepmothers. She helped me navigate my adolescence, grief, and rebellion, saving me from myself, as well as my life, many times along the way. She was always my anchor. Even after she married just shy of her eighteenth birthday and began to raise her two sons, we stayed connected however we could.

In 2004, with her boys now young men, one in the Marines, one settled in Syracuse after serving in the Air Force, she and her husband moved to North Carolina to escape the harsh Syracuse winters. Still, our friendship never wavered. We spoke on the phone regularly, and I made a few brief visits over the years. But when her husband died unexpectedly in 2013, I began making the trip annually. It was a trip I always looked forward to, just as I was that day in April 2022, waiting for the plane to take off.

My time with Julie is always so simple. We have our favorite little shops to visit, and we share conversations full of a lifetime of stories, family tales, and secrets. We laugh at memories of our youthful shenanigans and at the antics of the adults we'd become. We cried over our losses and celebrated our resilience. Life felt easy as we strolled through her neighborhood, lounged on her back patio, and floated in her pool under the warm, high sun. Mornings were quiet and peaceful, spent sipping coffee in her carport, rocking in chairs, letting the day unfold at its own pace.

This time was different. Every day, things started well, until one or two in the afternoon. Smack dab in the middle of a conversation or activity, I'd have to excuse myself and go lie down for an hour or so. Having lived alone for so long, I'd grown accustomed to needing time for myself when visiting friends. I told myself that's what I was doing, just taking some "me time." But honestly, I had no choice. Ever since the heart attack, I'd been carrying a portable blood pressure cuff, and each day, as I made it inside to the bed, my blood pressure would drop to anywhere between 86/58 to 75/50. I felt physically awful and emotionally powerless over my body—lightheaded, dizzy, weak, and completely unable to do anything but lie down.

Before I left to go back home to Syracuse, I called the cardiologist and moved my six-month follow-up appointment by a month. I understood that some things were part of a so-called "new normal," but collapsing in the middle of the day was not working for me. Something needed to change.

CHAPTER 22

KRIPALU

I still had more travel ahead. This time, I was making the two-hour, forty-minute drive to Kripalu, a yoga and wellness center nestled in the Berkshires of Massachusetts. I had planned to attend a weekend workshop led by Bessel van der Kolk, author of *The Body Keeps the Score*. I made these plans before the heart attack, and even though I wanted to cancel, I forced myself to go, determined to restore some normalcy in my life.

Kripalu turned out to be exactly what I needed. The sunshine, blue skies, and beautiful grounds were bursting with early spring blooms—multi-colored flowers pushing through the lush green lawns. The delicious organic foods easily fit into my food plan, and I found myself surrounded by a roomful of people eager to learn about and heal from trauma. The experiential activities took us deep into our psyches and our souls. At one point, I turned to Kate, a woman I had just met, and with the biggest smile on my face and a heart full of joy, I whispered loudly, "I belong!"

I belonged because Bessel spoke a language I understood, as did the people in the audience. I belonged because I didn't have to try to fit in, like forcing a square peg into a round hole. I belonged because this was exactly where I needed to be. I belonged simply because I was me.

On the second evening, as I rested in my room before dinner, I decided to check my phone. I'd had it on Do Not Disturb all day. There was a text from Aunt Annie, Mom's sister. It read simply, "Pam passed away."

I slumped to the floor and cried. I cried because I missed her in so many different ways, on so many different levels. I cried for the relationship we lost and never regained, believing we still had time. I cried for all the people who loved her deeply and for those who never had the chance to meet her. I cried because I was about to go do yoga and she couldn't. I cried for her husband and her devoted dog, Pearl—150 pounds of pure love, a mix between a great white Pyrenees and a poodle—who never left her side. I cried for her parents, Aunt Marge and Uncle Gary, who should never have had to watch their child die. I cried for her sister, Laura, who loved with a love so immense it defied words. And I cried especially for her sons, Sawyer (20) and Zane (18), knowing deep in my core the overwhelming pain that consumes you when your mom dies, no matter how old you are.

CHAPTER 23

THIRD FOLLOW-UP
APPOINTMENT

Driving home after a long weekend, navigating a whirlwind of emotions, I felt like I could take on the world. I was eager to apply the new insights I'd gained to my daily interactions, my relationships, and my own grief, trauma, and healing. There was a sense of urgency to live my life bigger, better, fuller, especially because Pam no longer could. Although, like so many retreats, the enthusiastic energy I carried home quickly faded as the world around me reasserted itself in familiar, frustrating ways.

Five months post-heart attack, I found myself back in Dr. Berkery's office. It was mid-afternoon, and my blood pressure was 85/62. I was told my heart was doing well. Sure, my EKG showed signs of a previous MI (myocardial infarction), which was expected, but my heart was strong, no longer sluggish. In fact, it looked as if nothing had happened. Yet, there I was, once again, asking the same question: *What is going on?*

Dr. Berkery and I reviewed everything. My medication, my

activity, my moods, my work. When did my blood pressure drop? Always in the afternoon, no other apparent pattern. Finally, we decided to stop my Metoprolol, a beta blocker that lowers both heart rate and blood pressure. My blood pressure naturally runs low, around 105/70, but I take the medication to keep my heart rate low. Dr. Berkery was hesitant to stop it and had me promise to closely monitor my heart rate. I laughed, because, trust me, I was paying close attention to everything heart-related.

Three days after stopping the medication, it was as if a light had turned on. I can't describe it any other way. It felt like I had been sitting in a dimly lit room, and someone walked in, flipped the switch, and suddenly, there was light. Not only did my blood pressure stop plummeting in the middle of the afternoon, forcing me to lie down, but the dullness I had been living with was gone.

Don't get me wrong, I didn't immediately leap into action and start doing all the things I thought were missing. But I was awake, aware, alert, and alive. My curiosity and enthusiasm began to peek out, tentatively and cautiously, like the Munchkins in *The Wizard of Oz* when Dorothy arrived, curious to see what was out there, yet unsure if what I was seeing was real or if it could be trusted.

CHAPTER 24

BABY STEPS

There were no dramatic changes I could pinpoint, just a series of subtle shifts carrying me forward. It was likely a combination of coming off the medication coupled with the sunshine and blue skies of Spring transitioning into Summer—a change that always has a profound effect on me.

As the weather improved, I began taking longer, more frequent walks. I monitored my heart rate closely, still hesitant to push it too high but slowly taking more risks, allowing it to climb just a bit higher for longer stretches. I had to begin to trust again. After all, what's the point of living if I remained a bystander, watching life from the sidelines, rather than stepping in and being a participant?

I started dancing around my apartment, rediscovering a joy I once loved. I moved with a wild mix of hip-hop, salsa, and contemporary styles that I created—a blend I'd never do in public but embraced fully in the privacy of my home. With the music loud and my body moving fast and free, I filled my spirit with the love that had been missing, as if reuniting with a long-lost friend. And at that moment, I was happy.

CHAPTER 25
THE POSSIBILITY
OF WRITING

Being off the Metoprolol and slowly emerging from the funk I had been living in, I couldn't help but wonder: Do people become depressed after a heart attack because of the physiological changes in their bodies? Or is it being forced to confront their mortality? Perhaps it's the medications prescribed to keep their hearts beating properly. I imagine it could be a combination of all three. For me, the fact that it was now May likely played a role in my brighter outlook after such a long, gray winter in Syracuse. Growing up in Syracuse, New York, it wasn't until twenty years ago that I realized I experience seasonal affective disorder, or S.A.D. Like clockwork, May brings a lightness to my world—mind, body, and spirit. Whatever the reason for this shift in perspective, I was grateful to be off the medication and thankful to be slowly rediscovering myself.

With Spring's arrival, energy coursing through my body, and a clearer mind, I began to dig deep, asking myself: What is my next

step forward? I decided to return to my writing, which I had abandoned for the last six months. Although, if I'm honest, it was never truly consistent or cohesive to begin with. I've been working on a memoir for most of my life, though it only started to take shape in 2020, at the onset of the COVID-19 Pandemic. I worked with a writing coach, Samantha Wallen, whose insight, compassion, and vision helped refine my focus and support my style. The story I felt compelled to tell revolved around my mother's death and the tumultuous, painful adolescence that followed. I wrote nearly 25,000 words, but then I stopped, allowing my resistance, procrastination, and doubt to reclaim their all-too-familiar place at the table.

CHAPTER 26

BREATHWORK

Over the next couple of years, I played with the memoir but couldn't seem to move it forward. Then, in June, just three weeks after I began to feel more awake and alive, I received a text from Meg. She urged me to check out an intense breathwork she had just experienced. Meg was the friend on the phone with me when my heart attack first began, as we discussed our next big workshop, goal, dream—something we've long since forgotten, but we remember it was huge. Like me, Meg is a feeler of feelings, a seeker of truth, both in herself and the world around her. Fittingly, her podcast is titled *Emotional Expedition with Meghan Thomas*. We met by happenstance at a kundalini yoga class, both of us attending on a whim, and instantly connected on our love of kundalini yoga, our grief from losing a parent young (she was five when her father died of a heart attack), and our love of Elizabeth Gilbert and Brene Brown.

Our friendship grew quickly and deeply, building a trust and respect that continues to connect us in the most profound ways today. So, when Meg tells me I need to check something out immediately, I find a way to make it happen. I couldn't attend the class she recommended the next day because I had to work, but she told me the name of the teacher who trained the woman leading her session. I signed up for a virtual Zoom class the following Sunday, where I was introduced to the man who would become my teacher in this amazing healing practice called Conscious Connected Breathwork: Jon Paul Crimi. His class opened me up to a direction I didn't even know I was searching for. He describes this type of breathwork as "One breathwork session is equivalent to 20 years of therapy without saying a word."

From Meg's first session and then mine, though our experiences were completely different, we both knew we wanted to be trained to facilitate this remarkable healing modality for others. I had heard stories of big emotional releases—crying, sobbing, uncontrollable laughter—and I wasn't surprised that mine wasn't like that. As open as I am about exploring and discussing emotions, physically, I tend to hold on tightly. Still, I showed up for Jon Paul's Zoom classes as often as possible, as well as doing the three-day replay he offers with each class. I didn't have the obvious emotional releases that I saw others experience though I often felt angry and impatient a few hours after the class in which I would dance it out around my apartment. What fascinated me was that even without a dramatic release, I could feel an ineffable shift inside—one that brought clarity and direction that kept me coming back for more.

At that point, two things were clear: I needed to finish my book, and I was signing up for the January Teacher Training in Denver, Colorado, to become a certified Breathwork facilitator. Before committing to the training, I needed to get cardiac clearance from Dr. Berkery—a reminder of how much my life had changed in the last year. It felt as if my life was no longer my own, and I needed permission to live it the way I wanted. Dr. Berkery was happy to clear me, glad to see me taking an interest in something positive.

In the months leading up to the training, I continued to practice Breathwork regularly, and I enrolled in a six-week online memoir program, *Overcoming the 6 Most Common Fears Memoirists Face*, with Brooke Warner and Linda Joy Myers. The class was a small taste of what they had to offer, and when it ended, I immediately signed up for their *Write Your Memoir in Six Months* program, which started a week before I headed to Denver for the Breathwork training. A little over a year had passed since my heart attack, and aside from an occasional glitch, everything finally felt like it was falling into place.

Meg and I walked into the conference room of the hotel with no expectations, just wide open to whatever might come. Thirty students from all over the country were there, eager to learn, release, and heal.

Being in a roomful of people instead of on Zoom was exhilarating, and I couldn't help but wonder: Is this where "it" will happen? Whatever "it" was. On the first day, although I felt open, I kept things close, reminding myself that I had invested a lot of time and money in these four days, and I needed to let go of any resistance I may be holding onto. On day two, Meg and I split up, sitting on different sides of the room. We partnered with whoever was next to us, encouraged to share our most intimate stories of grief and trauma with these new strangers, now confidantes, before starting a Breathwork session. My partner was a beautiful young woman in her early 30s named Barrett, her crystal blue eyes as clear as a perfect sunny day. I made a conscious choice to trust her with the deepest part of who I am so I could have the best possible experience.

I lay down on my yoga mat, ready to begin the open mouth breath, as she sat at my head, holding space for whatever might come up. Like a spin class, the music started, fast and loud, with Jon Paul, speaking into a microphone, encouraging us to breathe through our mouths. Two breaths in. One breath into the belly, one into the chest, followed by a gentle exhale. Over and over, the breath continued—no beginning or end. Circular, deliberate, focused. And then it happened: I felt the first tremble, unsure where it would lead. In the past, this is where I would've tried to take control, but not this time. This time, I stayed with the breath, trusting the process as it continued to build within me, bigger and faster, until it had nowhere to go but out. And there it was, it erupted—a release of emotions, coming out in tears, sobbing, even keening. Everything I had kept inside, even the things I thought were healed, poured out. Barrett stayed with me, gently holding my shoulders and arms, cradling my head, whispering words of love and encouragement, letting me know I was safe to let go of whatever needed to go.

At the end of the active breathing, we let out a primal scream. Until then, when I practiced at home, I couldn't scream from deep within, only from my throat, always coming out more like a cough. That day, after such a massive release, I screamed from the most cavernous part of myself with an intensity that touched my soul. As I screamed, my arms stretched wide, reaching toward the ceiling, and as the scream ended, my arms dropped to my sides, spread ea-gle. As my right arm hit the ground, I felt a sharp pain in my bicep; though I wasn't concerned, it held a small piece of my attention.

The pain in my arm persisted throughout the day, and I couldn't move it fully, but the lightness I felt from the release and the joy that filled me kept me from worrying. I intuitively knew it would be okay. That night, I had a dream. I was with my cousins, Pam and Laura. Laura, usually the center of attention, was in the background while Pam snuggled up against me, rubbing my arm up and down. I asked her why she was doing that, and she replied, "Just like when we were kids," as if this was something she had done long ago. It felt wonderful spending time with Pam, though I wasn't sure in the dream if I knew she had died. The next morning, unsurprisingly, my arm was completely pain-free with full range of motion restored.

Even with the two-hour time difference, I called my sponsor as always at our usual time, tripping over my words in my excitement, telling her in detail what occurred in the last 24 hours. She paused for a second before asking, "Why do you always dig so deep?"

"For the same reason you breathe," I responded with no hesita-tion, gratitude filling my voice as I added, "I have no choice."

I loved every moment of the four-day training. Over the years, I've been trained and certified in various modalities, some of which I still practice, if not professionally, definitely personally. I regularly practice Reiki, a Japanese technique for stress reduction, relaxation, and healing, as well as end-of-life and grief coaching. These are practices that are fully aligned with who I am and why I am here. Learning to facilitate Breathwork, as well as practicing it myself, has been life-changing. Of everything I have tried over the years, this simple open-mouth breathing technique has proven to be THE most effective and efficient way to release stored grief and trauma from my nervous system.

Before Meg and I even left for Colorado, we had already set the date and location to lead our first class, eager to share this with others. What we found, much like addiction recovery, is that while many people need this, and many want it, only those who are truly ready and willing to do the work will show up. I didn't know who would be ready to enter the proverbial arena, but I knew without a doubt that we were ready and willing to hold space for all those who did. We quickly learned that leading this level of raw, vulnerable healing is a profound privilege—to witness such bravery left us and them wanting more.

CHAPTER 27

FINDING MY WAY WITH MEMOIR

As I continued leading monthly classes, I deepened my personal Breathwork practice while navigating a six-month memoir course. Despite my best efforts, I stumbled, swerved, resisted, and procrastinated as I tried to gain traction with my book. Everything felt too big, too much. I had just started a new job before diving into the Breathwork training and the memoir class, and the shift from a minimalist lifestyle—working two to three days a week—to seven weeks of orientation, Monday-Friday, eight hours a day, was jarring. I realized this was a common workplace, but it had been a long time since I lived that way. I was left wondering: Where was the time to write, prepare my meals, do my recovery work, and breathe? I knew I had to find a way to make it work.

The first day of the memoir class felt like the first day of school. I was giddy with excitement I hadn't felt in ages. Armed with a new notebook and a fine-tip pen that made my handwriting flow, I sat at my laptop in my funky floral chair, ready to learn. As I logged into Zoom, I wondered about the teachers and my class-mates: What would they be like? Would I fit in? Did I belong? I told myself kindly, *Please don't let me dominate the space with my excitement and nerves like I used to.* As the class started, I heard a thought not my own, "Yes, Caron, you are right where you're supposed to be. You belong." And in that moment, I knew I did.

Years earlier, I was preparing to walk my grand puppy, an 18-pound Chihuahua-Pug mix named Lady Bark Ruffalo. She was so excited that she spun and swerved, making it almost impossible to put on her leash. Laughing, I asked her, "Why are you resisting something you love so much?" As the words left my mouth, they gave me pause. How often had I resisted things I loved or dreams I longed to fulfill?

This pattern followed me throughout my life—a story born in childhood. I was repeatedly told I wasn't living up to my potential, and that idea became embedded in my belief system. But what did "potential" even mean? And why did no one tell me what it was or how to reach it? There were moments when I broke through the lies I had mistaken for truth and accomplished significant things. Yet, even now, at 59, after years of overcoming the food and alco-hol that clouded the truth of who I am, peeling away the layers of false stories that no longer served me, I still found myself resisting, especially with my writing. As much as I wanted to write, the words formed in my mind, but I remained paralyzed, unable to bring them to the page.

I began to question whether it was the fear of failure or the fear of success holding me back. Failure was familiar territory—unpleasant, but something I had learned to navigate. With each failure, I picked myself up, brushed myself off, and moved on. Failure provided justifications: I didn't try, it didn't matter, I was kidding myself, it was a pipe dream. I used to think that I was a failure if I didn't know what I never learned or excelled at something immediately. Now, I see that my failures don't define me. And really, how could I fail if I never even stepped into the arena?

Success, on the other hand, felt foreign despite having achieved hard-earned goals. For much of my life, with every accomplishment I attained, for every bar I raised higher than before, I feared that others would expect me to maintain that standard—and I'd be exposed as a fraud. Balancing the need to be seen and heard with the discomfort of actually being seen or heard was a difficult dance.

I could spend hours, days, even months trying to figure out what is keeping me from moving forward, only to realize that *figuring it out* is just another form of procrastination. To figure out is not a tool, it is a distraction. In my experience, clarity comes in hindsight. I can't change my actions with thoughts, but I can change a thought with an action. If nothing changes, nothing changes, and the only way to move forward is to move forward. The only way to write a book is to write a book. It sounds simple, and it is, but when you're stuck in doubt and tangled in old stories, it's anything but easy.

Joining the memoir class was my first step forward. There, we were assigned writing buddies, carefully matched by our teachers based on what we were seeking in a partner. I wanted accountability and connection, and so did Joan.

It was an unexpected pairing, one I wouldn't have chosen on my own. It wasn't that Joan was 84 years old. That intrigued me. It was more that our stories, and how we told them, were so different. On paper, we couldn't be more different, but during our first Zoom meeting, I knew we were a perfect match. Joan's enthusiasm and curiosity thrilled me. Her passion for what she calls "dynamic aging" was infectious. And for me, what makes any relationship successful is open, honest communication that fosters a sense of safety, and I felt that with Joan immediately. It also wasn't lost on me that Joan was 11 months younger than my mom would be if she were still alive.

Even with the accountability and a partner I trusted, I still floundered with the direction of my writing. I knew the story that I wanted to tell, and every other week, I submitted my assignments and received positive feedback. And still, the struggle ran the show.

Since entering recovery and cultivating a relationship with a Higher Power, I've learned that when I struggle, it's because I'm trying to control the process, how things are done, and what the outcome should be. When I surrender and stop fighting, everything flows more naturally. Sure, obstacles and challenges still appear, but like floating down a river, I might bump into branches and rocks, yet they only nudge me forward. When I act as though I'm in charge, I may as well be swimming upstream.

At the end of the six-month class, Joan and I decided to keep each other accountable by meeting on Zoom every other week. I continued with my Breathwork practice, both facilitating and practicing on my own. Additionally, I've incorporated moon wishes into my routine, following Keiko's book *The Power Wish*. During the new and full moons, I use the tools she provides to manifest my deepest desires.

CHAPTER 28

SHARING MY HEART SONG

My vision for my memoir has always centered on my adolescence, focusing on the grief, anger, and betrayal I felt after my mother's death. The years between 13 and 18 were extremely self-destructive, intensely rebellious, deeply tumultuous, and filled with emotional turmoil—not just for me, but for everyone who loved me. I was like the Tasmanian Devil, spinning wildly and tearing down everyone and everything in my path. Especially myself. This was the story I had spent a lifetime preparing to tell. A story of grief, love, and resilience. Yet, despite my determination, something was holding me back. I continued to write, breathe, wish, and trust the process, unsure of what else to do.

As December 2023 arrived, two years after my heart attack and now 60 years old, I felt a spark inside of me—a clear vision of an idea that I knew I had to bring to life.

February is American Heart Month, a time dedicated to raising awareness about heart disease. This includes a day, the first Friday of the month, singled out called Go Red for Women, an initiative that highlights heart disease as the number one cause of death in women. I became energized, eager to focus on something rarely discussed but potentially lifesaving—how women present differently than men when having a heart attack.

Reflecting back to the day of my heart attack, this was one of my last of many thoughts before I called 911. *Women present differently than men.* But what did that really look like? I love to educate and inspire through personal experience. Through my work in a recovery program, I've seen firsthand the power of storytelling— how hearing others' experiences and sharing our own can create connection and understanding. Now, I was ready to share my cardiac story.

With two months to prepare, I started planning. My first thought was to reach out to a local publication, *Syracuse Woman Magazine.* Every February, the American Heart Association (AHA) sponsors an issue focused entirely on women's heart health.

I reached out to my friend Trina, who once worked for the AHA, even though she now lived in Italy. She was thrilled with the idea and immediately began brainstorming ways to get my story out there. While I waited for her to contact her former colleagues, I shared my plan with my writing buddy, Joan. Without hesitation, she invited me to write an article for her online magazine, *Dynamic Aging 4 Life Magazine,* which reaches more than 900 subscribers.

YES! The momentum was building. I began writing the article for *Dynamic Aging 4 Life Magazine,* which would also be featured in the *In Her Own Words* column in *Syracuse Woman Magazine.* I was curious: *Where else can I take this? How can I reach the largest audience possible to share this lifesaving information?*

During a full moon Power Wish group at the Center for Sound

and Ceremony, it hit me. I wrote down my wish, expressing gratitude as if it had already come true. *What if I could get the hospital where I work to support this educational initiative?* With over 3,200 employees and a strong community presence, this could have a huge impact.

I went home and immediately began drafting a letter to Bob Allen, Vice President of Communications and Governmental Affairs at the hospital. I could feel the spark expand as the plan was set in motion. It all made sense. I was born at Crouse Hospital, as were two of my children. I went to nursing school at Crouse, I worked at Crouse, my cardiologist was at Crouse, my life was saved at Crouse. This was happening.

Bob loved the idea and was just as excited as I was to move forward. He connected me with Laurie Clarke, Communications and Digital Media Manager. As I shared my story with her, I could feel her creative energy ignite. She was fully on board.

We started with an interview featuring Dr. Berkery and me for February's issue of *YourCare,* a Crouse publication designed to keep staff and the community informed about the latest services, programs, and health news. It is mailed out to more than 23,000 people in Central New York, along with 7,000 more reached via social media and many others finding it on the hospital website.

As the article took shape, Laurie scheduled a podcast interview for Crouse Healthcast, which then led to a two-minute video capturing the message beautifully. The video can be found at crouse. org/caron. We ended February with a Lunch and Learn event called Wellness Wednesday, featuring heart-healthy tips, snacks, games, and me sharing my story with attendees in person and over Zoom, followed by a Q and A.

I posted everything on my personal social media, feeling exposed and stirring up old insecurities that I was "too much." I worried that my intensity might scare people away. But this wasn't about me, I reminded myself. It is about the message. I intuitively knew that I had to keep going, sharing this message with everyone who would listen. So, I acknowledged the little "too much" gremlin that had been my companion for much of my life. With great love, compassion, and self-awareness, I asked it to take a seat in the back. This was too important to let the old stories drive this bus.

CHAPTER 29

THE STORY SHIFT

As I prepared for February, I continued working on my memoir, still focused on my adolescence and grief. Still, I kept running into a wall, painfully banging my head and getting nowhere. It was frustrating to have such flow and excitement in one area of my life while another part felt sludgy and heavy.

I still met with Joan on Zoom every couple of weeks to discuss our writing, though there were times I showed up empty-handed, unable to give her anything because all I could do was stare at a blank page. I found myself asking that awful question I had set aside for so long: *Who am I kidding, thinking I can write a book?*

Despite the negative self-talk, I stuck to it, remembering what I heard when I first came into recovery: It is only when I stay in the arena that the miracle knows where to find me. So dammit, I was going to keep showing up, ready, willing, and able when it did.

The first to come out as February rolled around was the article I wrote for Joan's online *Dynamic Aging 4 Life Magazine*. Joan and her team did a beautiful job with my story and the accompanying photos. Seeing this dream come to life filled me with deep gratitude and appreciation.

I sent the link to all the friends and family I could think of, as well as posted it on social media—not just because it was my story but because it was also my mother's. I believed in its necessity and felt a deep responsibility to share it. The feedback was encouraging and positive, but the most significant responses were from my aunts, Mom's two sisters.

Aunt Annie, who has always been willing to talk openly about my mom's life and death, responded with relief. She quickly texted me beautiful words of support, followed by a phone call. We spoke for nearly 30 minutes, honestly and intimately, sharing our memories of that long-ago Easter Sunday. She told me she had never been able to make sense of her sister's death, and now, almost 47 years later, something finally rang true for her.

"What if she died so that someday you could tell her story and possibly save lives? That would mean something. That could make sense of such a senseless death," she pondered aloud.

"If this helps you find peace, then so it is," I replied, tears welling up as my heart filled with gratitude.

Aunt Marge, who found it difficult over the years to talk about my mom's death, sent me a heartwarming text, thanking me for my service to humanity. For the first time, she shared intimate memories and added some family history, telling me that my great-grandmother and two great-aunts also died of heart attacks in their early 40s and 50s.

How did I not know this? Like a punch in the gut, I had to catch my breath. Anger built inside me as my body tensed and clenched—anger at the medical community, which I felt more and more often. Anger that Mom had to die too young, missing so much to come. Anger that Ellen and I, Marge and Ann, my dad, her friends—that we all had to live our lives without her. Anger at the senselessness of it all. How could Mom's doctors not explore her complaints more thoroughly, knowing her medical history?

As Aunt Marge and I texted back and forth, I realized I was no longer that thirteen-year-old girl, desperate for her love and approval. I was a woman, equal to her, standing in my own truth. She ended our text exchange with, *"Please keep writing and sharing your story."*

What I heard, despite the simplicity of the words, was: *YOU MUST SING IT FROM THE ROOFTOPS!*

In a blink of an eye, I experienced an intuitive knowing—a moment of instantaneous clarity. A visceral sensation swooshed through my body from head to toe. A whirlwind of energy made me want to jump for joy as I shook out my arms with an uncontrollable shiver. This is what happens when I feel a full body YES!

At that moment, I knew. *This* was the book I needed to write. *This* was the message I needed to share. For my mother and all the women misdiagnosed, their concerns discounted and brushed aside. For all those who have died unnecessarily, too scared to defy or question their doctors. For those unaware they have the right to be seen and heard. For those that defiantly advocate for themselves, only to be labeled crazy, hysterical, or emotional. This is for our mothers and daughters and sisters and aunts—for all the women we love. This is for you, and the time is now!

EPILOGUE
JUNE 20, 2024

My goal was to write this epilogue ten days ago, which would've been my mom's 87th birthday. But alas, as often happens, my plan took a detour, and instead, I found myself staring at a blank screen. It's no surprise that just as the heart attack occurred on the Winter Solstice, it feels right that the last page I write is on the Summer Solstice.

This wasn't the book I intended to write, but it is the book that needed to be written, opening the door for other books to follow.

My mother's death changed the trajectory of my life. Yes, I am still the Caron of my childhood, the same soul that I believe chose my parents to receive and learn the lessons that are mine. Yet, in my grief, anger, confusion, and adolescent immaturity, my choices became reckless, messy, and destructive.

I wish I wasn't the kind of person that needed a 2x4 smacking me in my head to get the point, but that's not my story. There is something to be said for finding purpose in one's pain, and thankfully, today, that 2x4 is lined with lamb's wool, caressing rather than swatting. And yes, this includes the heart attack.

Perseverance and resilience were never traits of mine I questioned, so after years of sludging, trudging, and seeking the truth of who I am, what my purpose is, and where I belong, here I am—connecting with you. I know I am never alone in this as we all sludge, trudge, and seek in our own individual ways, meeting each other where we are. Not where we think we should be or where others tell us we should be, but right here, right now, in all our beautiful messiness.

As much as I have learned along this journey, there's still much to discover. I will continue to seek, peeling back the layers of who I am. I will be as honest, open, and willing in the process, acknowledging, accepting, and hopefully improving what I find along the way.

On this day, 2 ½ years after a heart attack, three lessons have become clear to me:

STOP. LISTEN. ACT

STOP... In this busy world, in our busy lives—as women, mothers, caregivers, guides, trailblazers, wives, entrepreneurs, CEOs, pet owners, friends, daughters, employees, employers, humans, et cetera—we forget to stop. Someone, something, always comes first. Yes, we may do some *self-care*: jogging, yoga, meditating, taking a class, meeting a friend for coffee. As we do this, how often do we feel guilty or distracted by our ever-growing to-do list, thinking of what we *should* be doing instead?

We get so caught up in the world around us that we lose sight of the world within us. The *YOU* that is worthy of being seen and heard. The *YOU* that is complete just as you are. When we're so involved with the external that we no longer hear the internal, we miss what our bodies are desperately trying to tell us. We will miss the cues and the nudges and end up relying on that 2x4 hitting us like a homerun, hopefully not completely out of the park.

The message might be a reminder to breathe, to rest, to exercise, to dance. It might be recognizing that an ache or a pain has overstayed its welcome and needs attention. You will not be able to hear it if you don't take the time to stop.

For me, a weird sensation shooting up my jaw only to recede a few seconds later, and an odd ache at the base of my neck barely whispered heart attack. Because I paused everything around me and focused solely on my body, I became acutely aware it was trying to tell me something. What? I wasn't sure; however, by stopping, I put myself in a position to listen.

LISTEN… How often have we ignored our instincts? As children, we may have seen something wrong with our parents and when we asked about it, we were told they were fine, creating doubt in what we were seeing and feeling. We might have said we felt sad and were told to be happy. We might have shared that we were angry and told to be grateful. We may have been forced to hug that weird uncle at family functions, despite feeling uncomfortable. Maybe we were punished for expressing any feeling at all. We learned to doubt our intuitive knowing. Worse, we learned it didn't matter to begin with. Children often were seen and not heard. Who or what validated our thoughts, opinions, and voices? The doubt grew, and somewhere along the way, we came to believe the story that others must be right if we were so consistently wrong.

I worked as a triage nurse in two different offices, often listening to the same patients call time and again, desperate and scared, their symptoms worsening. I would approach the doctors with their concerns, often met with eye rolls and told that the patients were crazy, emotional, dramatic.

Women, BIPOC, and the LGTBQ+ community are notoriously dismissed and gaslit in healthcare. When professionals with years of education and training tell us it's anxiety, when they ignore our symptoms or fail to pursue answers more thoroughly, we begin to wonder: Maybe I am crazy.

Then there are the exceptional doctors who listen and dig for the answers, but their hands are tied by insurance companies that won't cover the costs of tests that could potentially save our lives, and we begin to wonder: Do I even matter?

With our sanity and our worthiness questioned, how do we learn to trust our instincts?

We practice. First, we practice with the small whispers, the little nudges, and as we listen, our faith in our instincts will begin to grow. Practice leads to progress, not perfection. Practice leads to better, and sometimes excellence.

ACT... Stopping long enough to listen to my body allowed me to face my fears, doubts, and disbelief. It was scary, but I decided I would rather take my chances of being wrong and possibly looking foolish than not act. The action I took was also an act of surrender. I had to let go of my ego, my fears, and my perceived control. I called 911.

It's funny; if a friend or loved one had been experiencing what I was, I would've had them call long before I did. To call for myself was the last resort.

Surrendering doesn't mean not participating in the experience. I still had choices. I chose to exaggerate my symptoms to the 911 operator. I chose to let others do their job. I chose to believe in a healthcare system that I often doubted.

Each action led to the next, whether it was mine or someone I put my trust in. At the end of the day, that action saved my life.

⇒⊦⊦⇐

I have learned to write down my questions before any appointment. I do this for two reasons.

1. To remember. Even if I think a question is too important to forget, in the moment, with nerves aflutter and the doctor's perceived hurry, the questions can disappear.
2. To remind the doctor that no matter how busy they are, I will not be rushed. My time is equally as valuable as theirs, and I deserve to be seen and heard.

I don't just ask the questions, I insist on answers. If I don't understand what I'm being told, it's not my fault. I am not stupid or inadequate. We can't know what we haven't learned. I ask them to explain until I understand.

I may have once gotten in my own way, not pausing long enough to hear what I intuitively needed or by not trusting what I heard.

We all have been born with an innate sense of self. I've spent years reclaiming my voice, and in doing so, I've become my greatest advocate. We have to be. We can't afford to wait for the right person, the right job, the right amount of money, or the right weight to believe in our worth.

No one knows my body as well as I do, and no one knows yours as well as you. The truth is, although we don't move through the world alone, no one or nothing is coming to save you. But you can. You are enough.

P.S. As I mentioned throughout the book, women may present differently than men when having a heart attack, but what might that look like?

Unlike the sudden, crushing chest or arm pain often associated with a heart attack, women's symptoms can be much more subtle and easily mistaken for other issues. For us, the pain may manifest as a vague discomfort in the neck, jaw, shoulder, upper back, or upper belly. It might not even feel like pain at all—sometimes, it's more like a flu-like sensation, accompanied by lightheadedness, dizziness, nausea, vomiting, or an overwhelming sense of fatigue that just doesn't make sense. These symptoms can be fleeting or persistent, but they are rarely the textbook signs we're taught to look out for.

With symptoms like these, symptoms we could easily dismiss or attribute to something else, why would we think of a heart attack? This is where "Stop. Listen. Act." comes in. This is the part I can't fully articulate. In the quiet presence of what I was experiencing, something told me to pay attention. A gut feeling, if you will. Something told me this was bigger than what was showing up.

At first, I wanted to ignore it, to rationalize what I was feeling as nothing serious. But ultimately, I couldn't. Eventually, I had to answer to that deeper knowing, to trust my instincts even when the evidence seemed murky. That, perhaps, is the most important takeaway. It's not just about recognizing the signs but listening to that internal voice telling you when something is off, even when none of what you're experiencing makes sense.

ACKNOWLEDGMENTS

My daughter, Lindsey Bortle, for making me a mom and inspiring me always to be the best version of me.

My son, Jake Field, for showing me a unique and interesting way of seeing the world. Listen to your heart song; I believe in your magic.

My sister, Ellen Moran, thank you for being on this journey with me—the challenges and celebrations, connected together like no other. I am so grateful for you!

My aunts, Marge Glowa and Ann Prowda, for always doing your best and encouraging me to get this story out there.

Meghan Thomas, for emboldening me to take the scary leaps and then magically becoming the net.

Gwen Minton, for always reminding me who I am and delighting in my so muchness.

Judy Pollman, from the beginning until now, your unwavering love and support have been home through it all.

Julie Gibbons, you may be far away, but you are always with me.

Julie Brown, the one who taught me that writing a book by following your intuitive knowing was even possible. (The Brownstone

Trilogy) I'm so grateful we made that promise to meet regularly for coffee and conversation so many years ago.

Helen McNeal, for offering me a home, a dog, and a warm place to land when I needed it most

Amy Lazzarini, for your quiet wisdom and dear friendship.

Joan Virginia Allen, my writing buddy, my sounding board, my friend. You inspire me daily to what it means to age dynamically.

Samantha Wallen, for challenging me in my writing and reminding me that I can be both a rebel and a rule follower.

My exuberant band of cheerleaders, Brenda Harrison, Meghan Boyce, Kasia Michalkow, Travis Field, Lisa Licitra, Janice Cushman, Valerie Braun, Jaime Weisberg, and Tracy Dando, thank you for believing in me (even when you had no idea what I was talking about) and always rooting for my success. Your support means everything!

Amy Assante, for your unflappable optimism and belief in my dream.

Sera McNaughton and Devorah Lewin, for exploring with me, *The Artist's Way, The Big Leap, and The War of Art.*

Brooke Warner and Linda Joy Myers, for teaching me memoir.

Dr. Bill Berkery, for truly hearing my fears and walking with me through one of the scariest times of my life. Your knowledge, kindness, and dedication will forever hold a place in my heart (no pun intended).

Dr. Anil George for saving my life, and Dr. John Ulahannan for assisting. Whatever word is 20 times bigger than grateful, THAT word!

All the staff on 4 North and the Cath Lab at Crouse Hospital, especially Megan Delaney, RN and Jo-Anne Furcinito, NP. I felt so well taken care of.

Jess Neiding and Laura Thorne, publishers extraordinaire at Wildebeest Publishing Company, LLC, for making this crazy, exhilarating, at times overwhelming adventure possible. Your encouragement and belief in me and the importance of my story have been life-changing! With the deepest of joy and gratitude, Thank you!

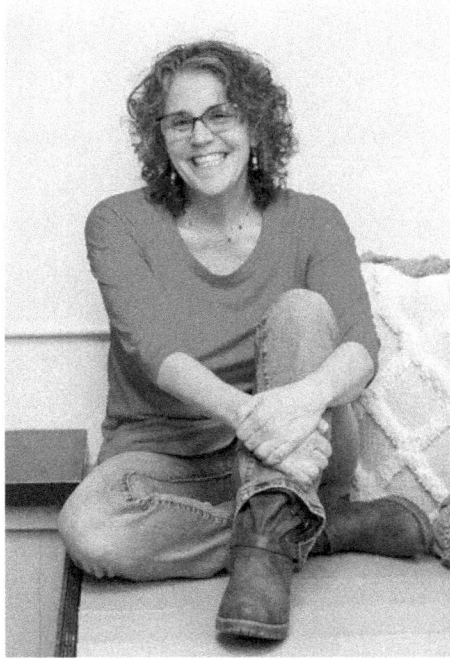

ABOUT THE AUTHOR

Caron, residing in Syracuse, NY is an RN, breathwork facilitator, and heart attack survivor, transforming life's challenges into stories of hope and healing. With warmth and insight, she shares wisdom with her TEDx talk, "Permission to Grieve," shaped by the sudden loss of her mother at 13. When she's not sharing her story and listening to others share theirs, Caron is enjoying music, reading, tossing a frisbee, or wandering the woods. She is fueled by family, friends, curiosity, and a passion for inspiring others to navigate the unexpected.